Emergency Medical Services:
an overview

Emergency Medical Services: an overview

Editors

Carl Jelenko, III, M.D.
Professor of Surgery
Director, Burn Investigation Laboratories
Medical College of Georgia
Augusta, Georgia

Charles F. Frey, M.D.
Director of Surgery
Martinez Veterans Administration Hospital
Martinez, California

Robert J. Brady Company
A Prentice-Hall Company
Bowie, Maryland 20715

76

Emergency Medical Services: an overview
First Edition

Copyright © 1976 by the Robert J. Brady Company
All rights reserved. This book, or any parts thereof, may not be used
or reproduced in any manner without written permission. For information, address the Robert J. Brady Company, Bowie, Maryland
20715.
Library of Congress Cataloging in Publication Data
Emergency medical services.

1. Emergency medical services. 2. Emergency medical services
—United States. I. Jelenko, Carl, 1931– II. Frey, Charles F.,
1929–
RA645.5.E47   362.1   76–7422

ISBN 0–87618–702–5

Prentice-Hall International, Inc., London
Prentice-Hall of Australia, Pty., Ltd., Sydney
Prentice-Hall of India Private Limited, New Delhi
Prentice-Hall of Japan, Inc., Tokyo
Prentice-Hall of Southeast Asia (Pte.) Ltd., Singapore

Printed in the United States of America

76 77 78 79 80 81   10 9 8 7 6 5 4 3 2 1

Contents

Contents

Contributors

Curtis P. Artz, F.A.C.S., Professor and Chairman, Department of Surgery, Medical University of South Carolina, Charleston, South Carolina

Don M. Benson, M.D., F.A.C.S., Assistant Professor, Department of Anesthesiology, Canton-Aultman Hospital, Canton, Ohio

William F. Bouzarth, M.D., F.A.C.S., Professor of Neurosurgery, University of Pennsylvania Hospital, Philadelphia, Pennsylvania

Neil L. Chayet, Attorney at Law, Boston, Massachusetts

Robert H. Dailey, M.D., Chief, Department of Emergency Medicine, Valley Medical Center, Fresno, California

Lionel L. Drage, Director, Emergency Medical Services, Intermountain Regional Medical Program, University of Utah, Salt Lake City, Utah

Paul A. Ebert, M.D., F.A.C.S., Professor and Chairman, Department of Surgery, Cornell Medical Center, Duke University, Durham, North Carolina

Charles F. Frey, M.D., F.A.C.S., Director of Surgery, Martinez Veterans Administration Hospital, Martinez, California; Vice Chairman, Department of Surgery, University of California, Davis

Paul W. Gikas, M.D., Staff Pathologist, Veterans Administration Hospital; Professor of Pathology, University of Michigan Medical School, Ann Arbor, Michigan

Ake Grenvik, M.D., Professor of Anesthesiology; Director, Division of Critical Care Medicine; Director, Presbyterian-University Hospital Intensive Care Unit, Pittsburgh, Pennsylvania

William T. Haeck, M.D., Emergency Physician, Jacksonville, Florida

John M. Howard, M.D., F.A.C.S., Professor of Surgery, Crozer-Chester Medical Center, Upland-Chester, Pennsylvania

Francis C. Jackson, M.D., F.A.C.S., Professor and Chairman, Department of Surgery, University of Texas Tech School of Medicine, Lubbock, Texas

Martin Keller, M.D., Ph.D., Professor of Preventive Medicine, Division of Community Health, Ohio State University, Columbus, Ohio

Allen P. Klippel, M.D., F.A.C.S., Director, Emergency Medicine Services for the City of St. Louis; Director, Emergency Department, St. Louis County Hospital, St. Louis, Missouri

Ronald L. Krome, M.D., F.A.C.S., Associate Professor of Surgery, Department of Surgery, Wayne State University School of Medicine; Director, Emergency Department, Detroit General Hospital, Detroit, Michigan

Sam Landrum, M.D., F.A.C.S., General Surgeon, Ft. Smith, Arkansas

A. James Lewis, M.D., Assistant Professor and Director, Cardiac Care Unit, Department of Medicine, Harbor General Hospital, Torrance, California

Milton N. Luria, M.D., Professor of Medicine, University of Rochester School of Medicine, Rochester, New York

Karl G. Mangold, M.D., Vice-President, American College of Emergency Physicians; Director, Department of Emergency Medicine, Vesper Memorial Hospital, San Leandro, California

James D. Mills, M.D., Emergency Physician, Alexandria, Virginia

John H. Morton, M.D., F.A.C.S., Professor of Surgery, University of Rochester School of Medicine, Strong Memorial Hospital, Rochester, New York

Brig. Gen. Donald G. Penterman (Ret.), Special Assistant to the Chancellor, University of Nebraska Medical Center, Omaha, Nebraska

Marie Piantanida, M.A., Administrative Specialist, Western Pennsylvania Medical Program, Pittsburgh, Pennsylvania

Andrew C. Ruoff, III, M.D., F.A.C.S., Associate Professor of Surgery, Department of Surgery, University of Utah, College of Medicine, Salt Lake City, Utah

Peter Safar, M.D., Professor and Chairman, Department of Anesthesiology; Coordinator, Multidisciplinary Critical Care Medicine Program, University of Pittsburgh, Pittsburgh, Pennsylvania

Daniel J. Scott, Jr., M.D., F.A.C.S., Orthopedic Surgeon, Memphis, Tennessee

John M. Waters, Director, Public Safety, Department of Public Safety, City of Jacksonville, Jacksonville, Florida

Preface

Presented in this book are the best judgments of twenty-eight national leaders and thinkers in the rapidly evolving effort to improve the organization and delivery of emergency care to the acutely ill and injured in the United States. These individuals have been innovators of change and effectors of progress in this effort; none are merely observers or historians.

Most of these individuals have become "experts" through their continued and intense study and involvement in efforts to improve emergency health services; most were not originally trained in public health, epidemiology, local or state politics, or in the sciences of organization and cybernetics which have become so much a part of the contemporary emergency health service scene. Instead, most were physicians of all stripes and specialties and/or military personnel.

Regardless of his professional background, each had a sense of community responsibility, vision, and idealism that enabled him to recognize the need to improve care to the acutely ill and injured. He saw the deficiencies in current emergency care, not so much as the result of a lack of skill and technology necessary to deliver such care, but rather as the result of a lack of planning, coordination, and organization of those elements necessary to effectively care for this patient population.

As a group, the authors and contributors met all of the existing stumbling blocks as they pursued their efforts to develop a *system* for appropriate delivery of emergency medical care. The authors detail these pitfalls, often with whimsy and humor. It is not surprising that pioneers grow through a process of trial and error, and it is not unexpected that medical professionals are naive about the political process. It is anticipated that early inexperience should be manifest in many of the skills in systems design, communications technology, new medical devices, and other such areas. However, these individuals were able to perceive information outside of their special fields of professional activity with great adaptability and to develop successfully new skills, most of which are detailed in this volume. The reader will find a concise presentation of the important concepts essential to the improvement of emergency medical services and to the understanding of elements contributing to an emergency medical services system. Whether the reader is a physician, nurse, emergency medical technician, hospital administrator, areawide health planner, public health official, or student, we believe the cumulative experiences in the pages that follow will be invaluable.

Throughout the literature on emergency medicine and emergency health care delivery, there is frequent use of jargonistic phrases. This book is not without the same defects. Nomenclature changes from day to day, from author to author, and from individual to individual. Thus, *allied health personnel* is a term used to mean and to be equivalent to paramedical personnel, physiotherapist, occupational therapist, and even, at times, nurses. In a similar manner, the term *crash injury management course* is equivalent to first responder's course, and *health services agency* is the same as comprehensive health planning. It may well be that other jargon will be used for those and for other terms throughout this book. The reader is requested to interpret this jargon using his own biases and neologisms. In his chapter on coronary care (chapter 4) Dr. A. J. Lewis comments on the Mobile Life Support Unit (MLSU), comprising the Mobile Coronary Care Unit (MCCU); and the Mobile Intensive Care Unit (MICU). He also describes and defines the Stationary Life Support Unit (LSU). Drs. Grenvik and Safar, in their chapter on critical care medicine (chapter 23), describe the Mobile Intensive Care Unit (MICU). These terms appear to the editors to be equivalent.

To the author group we bow deeply in admiration and gratitude.

Carl Jelenko, III, M.D.

Charles F. Frey, M.D.
June, 1976

Emergency Medical Services:
an overview

I

Overview

Curtis P. Artz

1

Acute Illness and Injury in the United States

Acute illness has become a primary health problem as a result of the rapid growth of the United States and the increased demands of its citizens for improved medical care. The public recognizes that medicine has advanced to such a degree that improved care for acute illness and injury is an obtainable objective. Developing an improved system of care should be the responsibility of the consumers as well as of the providers. The people of this country must be made aware of the enormity of the acute illness and injury problem so that they can be motivated to assist in the provision of better care for this aspect of the health needs of the United States.

Accidental injury is a major challenge to modern medicine. In the United States in 1972 there were 52 million injuries, 117,000 deaths, and 420,000 permanent disabilities at a national cost of $32.3 billion. These figures make accidental injury a monumental health issue. Automobile accidents accounted for about half the injuries, home accidents for 24%, and injuries at work for 12%. These men, women, and children occupied more hospital beds than did heart patients and four times more beds than did cancer patients. Accidental injury is the fourth leading cause of death in the nation and the leading cause of death for the population of the ages 1–37.

Many people do not realize that accidents not only damage the outer body but also produce internal injuries. For example, a study of 950 autopsies of accident victims reveals that, in 38% of those who died following a fracture of the hip, the primary cause of death was actually pulmonary embolism. Yet, in a large number of similar patients who had not been autopsied, pulmonary embolism was the recorded cause of death in only 2%. This study exemplifies the dearth of knowledge concerning trauma. If autopsies were performed in all cases of death due to trauma, they would provide an invaluable source of information that is needed to establish a basic defense against this killer.

Today in the United States myocardial infarction kills 400,000 annually. The percentage of deaths from this cause is higher in rural areas than in urban areas. The inadequacies of communications systems, ambulances, ambulance equipment and training of ambulance personnel, and the lack of coordination between transportation systems and hospitals capable of providing care to the acutely ill and injured are universal but are especially notable in rural areas.

Death from traffic injuries has increased annually. Ten thousand more were killed in 1965 than in 1955, and this trend still continues. Seventy percent of the motor vehicle deaths occurred in rural areas and in communities with populations under 2,500. In 1 year alone vehicle accidents killed more people than the United States lost in the Korean War. In the past 60 years more Americans have died from accidents than from combat wounds in all wars. During wartime, deaths from accidents always exceed battle deaths. In World War II, U.S. battle deaths totaled 292,000; accidental civilian deaths during the same period in the United States alone was 450,000. Even more military personnel die from accidents than from combat during a period of national involvement. For example, in Vietnam from 1962 to 1965 there were 1,557 combat deaths, while there were more than 10,000 deaths from accidents in the armed services during this same period.

The care of accident victims imposes a staggering load on physicians, paramedical personnel, and hospitals. Approximately one out of every four Americans suffers an accident of some type each year. Many are treated at home and work, but most receive medical attention in a physician's office or in the outpatient or emergency departments of hospitals. It is estimated that in 1965 more than 2 million victims of accidental injury were hospitalized. They occupied 65,000 hospital beds for 22 million bed days and received the services of 88,000 hospital personnel. This number exceeds that of bed days required to care for the 4 million babies born each year or to care for all heart patients, and it is more than four times greater than that required for cancer patients.

Almost half of the deaths of children (ages 1–15) in the United States are the result of trauma, compared with approximately one death in ten resulting from injury in the total population. Death of a child is tragic, but crippling injuries and the associated needs for rehabilitation constitute a far greater percentage of resources and personnel required. In addition, the economic loss to society that results from the termination of work productivity when a child is seriously handicapped is relatively expensive when compared with such injuries in adults. Because of the limited reserves of small children and the rapidity with which they deteriorate, transportation of the injured child assumes increased importance.

It is well to get a relative view of the work-injury total. In 1912 an estimated 18,000 to 21,000 workers died at a time when the United States was producing a $100 billion gross national product. In 1968, with a work force doubled in size and producing more than eight times as much as in 1912, there were only 14,300 occupational deaths. Since 1912 the number of work deaths per 100,000 population has been reduced 67%. This reduction speaks well for American industry. Our present occupational problem may be a formidable one, but it is under better control than it was 50 years ago.

The prominence of deaths from accidents is being recognized as a phenomenon of the twentieth century. In 1900 accidents ranked fourth as the total cause of deaths among young people, but by 1940, while deaths from accidents remained between 40 and 60 per 100,000 population, there was a steady drop in the death rate from other major causes, so that accidents, for the first time, exceeded all other causes of death in this age group.

While the number of deaths from accidents per 100,000 population or per million miles of vehicular travel decreased during this time, the increase in population and in automobiles has resulted in an increase in the absolute death rate in all categories. Ever increasing horsepower coupled with an unchanging degree of human error exceeded the rate of our willingness or ability to incorporate safety features into our automobiles.

5

The trend in accident death rates of children has been downward since 1900, but the proportion of absolute childhood deaths due to accidents has been increasing. In 1966, four out of every ten children who died in the United States were victims of trauma. Injuries have been the leading cause of death of children for over 10 years. Haller has reported that more than 100,000 children are permanently crippled in the United States each year by accidents, and another 2 million are temporarily incapacitated by injury.[1] This number is in addition to approximately 13,000 deaths from accidents between the ages of 1 and 14.

COST

Each year it is estimated that over 500 million days of restricted activity are the result of accidental injury, which represents nearly 20% of the restricted activities from all medical causes. Short-term conditions having restricted activity due to accidental injury even exceed those due to the common cold. The tangible economic loss expressed as cost and expenses from accidents is estimated by the National Safety Council to be over $22 billion per year. Part of this loss is visible, but much of it is not apparent except to the victims, their families, medical and hospital personnel, lawyers, employers, courts, and the insurance companies.

It is impossible, however, to measure the full economic impact of trauma. There are many injuries, particularly off the job, that are never recorded, and many of those that are recorded do not include some of the indirect costs that result. It must also be remembered that some degree of human suffering accompanies every injury, and many of them bring a tragic aftermath. About $2 billion is now paid annually to claimants from the private workmen's compensation insurance industry.

Of the more than 2 million work injuries that occurred in 1968, 14,300 proved fatal and 90,000 resulted in some permanent impairment. The National Safety Council estimates the cost of these work injuries at 245 million lost man days and nearly 8 billion lost dollars.

Disabling injuries account for a far greater share of total cost than do fatalities. The National Safety Council reported 11 million such injuries in 1968, including only those injuries that prevented the performance of usual activities for a full day. The council's breakdown on the disabling injuries in 1968 is (1) home accidents, 4.5 million; (2) public non-motor vehicle accidents, 2.5 million; (3) motor vehicle accidents, 2 million; and (4) work accidents, 2 million. Table 1.1 gives an indication of cost per fatal injury.

Schlueter states that there is a major economic impact with many

Table 1.1.   Fatal Accidents: 1968

Type of accident	Annual number of fatalities	Average cost per death
Home accidents	28,500	$ 75,000
Public non-motor vehicle accidents	20,500	$ 75,000
Motor vehicle accidents	55,200	$ 38,700
Work accidents	14,300	$275,000

types of injuries.[3] He cites cost as follows: (1) fracture of the neck of the femur, $19,600; (2) fracture of both heels, $19,500; (3) penetrating eye wound, $11,900; and (4) fracture of the wrists, $6,900.

Many times there are mental as well as physical complications of injury. Sometimes injury is complicated by hysterical symptoms, commonly referred to as traumatic neurosis. One especially susceptible group seems to be unmarried women over 30 who are involved in assembly work requiring speed and dexterity and who suffer hand and arm injuries. These individuals tend to develop strong fears that their dexterity is irrevocably lost and that their usual productive lives are at an end.

Unlike some diseases whose symptoms can be described but are without cures, the remedies that will improve the care of the acutely ill and injured are known and can be purchased at a reasonable price. The potential for salvage of lives lost unnecessarily in the United States has been estimated by Huntley to be 22,500 for the 120,000 killed from accidents and 35,000 for the 400,000 dying from myocardial infarction each year.[2] The cost of improving hospital emergency medical service systems to annually salvage 55,000 persons now dying from acute illness and injury has been estimated to be $2 billion or 2.5% of the present $80 billion health budget.

EMERGENCY MEDICAL SERVICES

Inadequate emergency medical care is a national problem that has recently come into the limelight. The most critical needs are (1) communications in an emergency; (2) prompt and proper rescue handling; (3) swift and careful transportation of victims; and (4) adequate emergency care at the hospital.

It has been estimated that 20,000 accident victims die needlessly every year because of deficiencies in our emergency medical services. The Automobile Association of America estimates that 25,000 people are permanently disabled each year by inadequately trained ambulance and rescue crews.

Estimates place the number of ambulances in use throughout the nation at about 45,000; approximately one for 5,000 people. There are about 7.5 million ambulance calls answered each year. In the southeastern section of the United States, estimates of the number of ambulance calls made and answered to emergencies run from 100,000 a year in Tennessee to 600,000 a year in Florida. Considering the great number of calls, the disturbing thing is that only a small percentage of the ambulances meet recommended standards for design and equipment. Less than half are equipped with two-way radios, and only a few have telemetry equipment. The Ambulance Association of America has estimated that 25,000 persons are permanently injured or disabled each year by untrained ambulance attendants and rescue workers.

PREVENTION

The long-term solution to the injury problem is prevention. The major responsibility for accident prevention rests not with the medical profession but with the educators, industrialists, engineers, public health officials, and private citizens. Although the physician is concerned primarily with increasing survival and lessening disability of victims after accidents occur, there are many ways in which the medical profession can help to prevent accidents. These include the detection and reporting of health hazards in the environment and calling attention to dangerously designed vehicles, appliances, houses, and public buildings. A reporting system must be designed to identify the types of accidents and the roles of human behavioral, physical, emotional, and mental defects; of acute and chronic illness; and of alcohol and drugs in accidents.

Man has a persistent tendency to tamper with his environment and to live in it without sufficient attention to the consequences. Complexity of the public health problems today is largely a result of man's alteration of his environment. The greatest threat lies in expansion of our intellectual activity itself. We are pressured by our own biologic success. Although newspapers may highlight deaths due to tornados in the Midwest or hurricanes in the South, the grim fact is that on any weekend more persons are killed on the highways by motor vehicles than are killed by the total forces of nature. A major obstacle to understanding this situation has often been the tendency to regard a given problem, whatever its nature, as unconquerable. This tendency has been the case with accidents. Public opinion has tended to regard accidents as unfortunate occurrences to be accepted as inevitable.

A major national educational program is needed in the area of accident prevention. Now, with the latest research, the two dimensions of the problem of traumatic injuries will only come through the development of a system of national injury data gathering and analysis. For instance, in 1954 there was an interscholastic athletic association that gained national attention for the data it gathered on high school athletic injuries, pinpointing mouth injuries as a major problem in high school football. The identification of 356 mouth injuries incurred from high school football led to the requirement of improved face guards and helmets; mouth injuries began dropping sharply. In 1967, with twice as many players, injuries of this type were reduced from 356 to only 97. As we gather more information about injuries we can warn individuals and suggest certain protection.

The important fact is that some injuries take a much greater toll than do others. Those taking a heavy toll are known as the "vital few," which is based upon the well-known statistical concept that in any body of data only a relatively small number of cases are truly significant. A Wisconsin insurance company has shown, in applying this concept to industrial accidents, that one-third of the total injuries account for 90% of the cost. In fact, 2% generate 50% of the cost. Such information permits management to focus its efforts in the areas of safety most likely to produce the quickest and greatest reduction in suffering and in economic loss.

About $2 million is spent each year for trauma research by the National Institutes of Health. This amount is only a pittance for research concerning the fourth leading cause of death in the United States. Recent studies indicate that the National Institutes of Health and the Public Health Service expend only 50 cents for each of the ten million persons disabled by accidental injury, while research funds in the amounts of $220 and $76 are expended for each of the estimated 540,-000 cancer cases and 1.4 million cardiovascular cases respectively. In the overview of acute illness and injury, it is obvious that more research money must be provided in this category.

THE REAL PROBLEM

Unlike other great killers, there has not been the unified response to trauma deaths that has brought the other killers under control and reduced their toll. The reason for this difference is the clear objective that goes with finding a biologic cause of disease and then the means of prevention. This is not the case with accidents. Prevention is immensely diffused, requiring not only medical research but also engineering and design research and control of many phases of industry and transportation as well as legislation.

The problem of trauma in this country and elsewhere is far more immense than is commonly realized. Most of us see it only in bits and pieces, brief accounts of accidental injury to individuals in their homes, on the streets, or at their jobs. Few of us comprehend the tragic and far-reaching aftermath of many such injuries, and few of us can guess what it all totals as irretrievable losses to individuals, families, nations, and the society at large. Traumatic injury is termed the neglected disease of a neglected epidemic of modern society.

The study and treatment of trauma are not just neglected. In many instances they are actively suppressed. For too many years, too many people have considered it such an undignified, untidy, and heterogenous subject that it was unworthy of intellectual effort. We have heard this opinion from both academic and government sources, again demonstrating that lack of vision and understanding is not confined to any one component of society. Syphilis was also a difficult and distasteful subject, but that did not prevent the initiation of massive public health service and university programs to control the disease. Cancer is also a heterogenous disease of multiple etiology and diverse manifestations and complications, but this has not discouraged the multitude of workers in this field.

The protean nature of trauma is precisely what makes it such a challenge. There is something significant in this subject for every biomedical related scientist from the most basic macromolecular chemist to the most applied industrial engineer. There are highly relevant problems for behavioral scientists, biomechanical engineers, internists, pathologists, economists, hospital administrators, pharmacologists, computer scientists, as well as physicians.

The challenge of acute illness and injury lies before the American people. It is hoped that physicians will take the leadership in improving this aspect of health care. But the emphasis is made that physicians alone cannot accomplish what needs to be done and that an overall effort from all our citizens is necessary and desirable.

REFERENCES

[1] Haller JA, Jr.: Problems in children's trauma. J Trauma 10:269, 1970
[2] Huntley H: The first hours are critical in medical emergencies. JACEP 1 (2):13–16, 1972

[3] Schlueter CF: Some economic dimensions of traumatic injuries. J Trauma 10:915–920, 1970

SUGGESTED READING

Accidental death and disability: The neglected disease of modern society. Washington, National Academy of Sciences, National Research Council, 1966

Artz CP, London PS, Bohler J, Hampton OP, Jr.: Panel discussion: General organization for trauma care and study. J Trauma 10:1012–1024, 1970

Jelenko C III (ed): Proceedings Second Annual Meeting, University Association for Emergency Medical Services. May 12–13, 1972, Washington, Division of Emergency Health Services, Public Health Services, Department of Health, Education, and Welfare

Proceedings First Regional Conference, Emergency Medical Services. May 2–3, 1972, Atlanta, Georgia. U.S. Department of Health, Education, and Welfare, Public Health Service, Health Services and Mental Health Administration

Shires T: Initial care of the injured patient. J Trauma 10:940–948, 1970

Stone FL: Report: Conference on Trauma, Public Health Service publication, No. 1565, Washington, National Institute of General Medical Sciences, 1966

Paul W. Gikas

2

The Accident Problem

The 1973 edition of *Accident Facts* published by the National Safety Council defines accident as "that occurrence in a sequence of events which usually produces unintended injury, death, or property damage."[1] In 1972, 117,000 persons were killed in the United States in accidents. Table 2.1 depicts the major categories of accidental deaths during that year.

Accidents are exceeded only by heart disease, neoplasms, and cerebral vascular diseases as a major cause of death in the United States. From age 1 to 38 years, accidents are the leading cause of death. Fourteen thousand one hundred persons were fatally injured in non-motor vehicle accidents while at work, and 26,800 persons were killed in

Table 2.1. Major Categories of Accidental Death*

Type of accident	Number of deaths
Motor vehicle	56,600
Falls	17,400
Drowning	7,600
Fires	6,800
Poisoning by gas, vapors, liquids, and solids	5,300
Suffocation	3,900
Firearms	2,400

* Modified from Accident Facts, Chicago, National Safety Council, 1973.

non-motor vehicle accidents associated with the home. A total of 11,-500,000 persons were non-fatally injured in accidents in 1972, with 2,100,000 injuries occurring in motor vehicle accidents. It is obvious from these statistics that motor vehicle crashes account for the largest number of accidental deaths.[1] These are categorized in Table 2.2.

Since the highway is the major arena of accidental violence in our society, discussion will concentrate on pathogenesis of injuries to occupants of cars and trucks involved in crashes.

Table 2.2. Major Categories of Motor Vehicle Fatal Accidents*

Type of vehicle	Number of deaths
Passenger cars	35,100
Pedestrians	10,700
Trucks	5,500
Motorcycles	2,500
Snow machines	156
Commercial buses	100
School buses	50

* Modified from Accident Facts, Chicago, National Safety Council, 1973.

MOTOR VEHICLE ACCIDENTS

Injuries sustained in motor vehicle accidents present a major challenge to the personnel involved in the care of the victims. An understanding of the mechanism of injury can be of considerable aid to the emergency medical technician and physician. Specific injury patterns are characteristic of certain crash circumstances, and knowledge of this relationship can raise the index of suspicion of the examiner, thus enhancing considerably the correct diagnosis and subsequent therapy.

Mechanical energy is utilized in the production of the injury. The forces involved in injury production result from deceleration or in some instances acceleration of the individual. The magnitude of the forces of deceleration or acceleration are related directly to the square of the change in velocity of the person and inversely related to the stopping distance of the individual.[6] These relationships can be expressed by the formula

$$g = \frac{V^2(\text{miles per hour})}{SD(\text{feet}) \times 30}.^1$$

The units of gravity that express the force of deceleration or acceleration are referred to as g in the formula. The reduction in velocity of the individual from the speed at which he was traveling to zero as the result of the impact is referred to as V in the formula.[1] The stopping distance *(SD)* refers to the distance over which this change in velocity occurs.

In situations of acceleration the velocity change refers to the increase in the person's velocity; the distance over which this change occurs is comparable to the stopping distance. In a crash involving a motor vehicle, the stopping distance is produced by deformation in the vehicle as well as deformation in the object with which the vehicle collides. The stopping distance is also referred to as crush distance, and in some instances may amount to several feet.

This crush is very beneficial to the occupant of the vehicle because of the inverse relationship between this crush or stopping distance and the decelerative forces produced by the crash. It is important to realize, however, that the occupant of the vehicle must be restrained in the vehicle in order to take advantage of the stopping distance afforded by the deformation of the vehicular structure. If the individual is not fastened to the vehicle by an active or passive restraint system, in a forward collision he continues to move forward at essentially the velocity at which the vehicle was traveling prior to the impact. After the deformation to his vehicle occurs, he then decelerates against some forward structure in his vehicle. The deformation produced in the interior surface of the vehicle that he contacts is his stopping distance. This contrasts the much greater stopping distance afforded by the anterior crush in the front of the vehicle. The area of the interior of the vehicle with which the body comes in contact in the so-called "second collision" influences the type and severity of bodily injury sustained.

The following examples illustrate the tremendous differences in decelerative forces resulting from changes in stopping distance. In utilizing the above formula, it becomes apparent that in an automobile involved in a forward crash at 35 miles per hour, sustaining a forward crush of 2 feet, the resulting deceleration is 20 g. If the occupant of this vehicle were fastened to the vehicle with an upper torso and lap-belt restraint system he would sustain approximately the same amount of g. However, an unrestrained occupant in the same crash decelerating against an instrument panel producing a deformation in the panel of only 2 in. would sustain 245 g. For an individual weighing 100 lb., this would mean a difference of sustaining 2,000 lb. of force in the first example and 24,500 lb. of force in the second example. The first example is well within the limits of survivability, whereas the second would be fatal.

From a study of 235 necropsy records by the author and his colleagues of persons fatally injured in automobile crashes, it was apparent that the majority of the victims had sustained injuries to more than one body area, and the head was the site most frequently injured.[9] This increased frequency of fatal head injuries in a series of crash fatalities reflects the vulnerability of the head to injury as well as the poor salvage potential for serious brain injuries.

In a previously reported study, ejection and the second collision within the vehicle emerged as the major events in the pathogenesis of fatal injuries to automobile occupants.[8] Ejection from an automobile involved in a crash occurs through open doors, side windows, windshield, and open roofs. As noted earlier the second collision involves the contact of the occupant with a surface within the interior of the vehicle. In the study referred to, 27% of the deaths resulted from ejection. In addition there were 14% who sustained fatal injuries from a second collision within the vehicle prior to being ejected. Although fire and submersion as the result of vehicular crashes are relatively uncommon events, they increase the potential for fatalities, and they make salvage attempts much more difficult.

The pathogenesis of injury to occupants of automobile and truck crashes and the principles of injury prevention are exemplified in some crashes described below.

Case 1.   A small car was occupied by a driver who lost control of the vehicle and caused it to roll over. The driver was ejected from one of the doors, which had opened (Fig. 2.1). The victim was subsequently crushed by the vehicle and died as the result of suffocation. Necropsy revealed broken ribs and vomitus in the trachea. It is obvious that this fatality could have been prevented if the door of the vehicle had remained closed and the occupant had been restrained by a seat belt.[7]

Case 2.   A recent model car collided with the rear of a large truck, which was attempting a U-turn in front of the forward-moving car on an expressway. The contact area was to the right front of the automobile which resulted in a rearward displacement of the right posterior corner of the hood through the windshield into the right guest passenger area (Fig. 2.2). This particular hood design, which has been popular in American vehicles since 1969, has an upward flare to its posterior margin, thus covering the windshield wipers in their resting position. This particular styling feature allows the hood to intrude through the windshield in this type of crash.

The car was occupied by a driver and a right front passenger; both were wearing lap seat belts. The driver sustained a minor facial injury, apparently as the result of his flexing forward over the lap belt and striking the steering wheel. The right front passenger, however, sustained a fatal head injury when she flexed forward over the lap belt and sustained a second collision with her face striking the axelike end of the hood, which had penetrated the windshield (Fig. 2.3). This is an example of a second collision between an occupant and a portion of the vehicle that has intruded into the occupant space as the result of the crash. The lap seat belt alone obviously was insufficient to protect against this type of second collision. It is questionable whether an

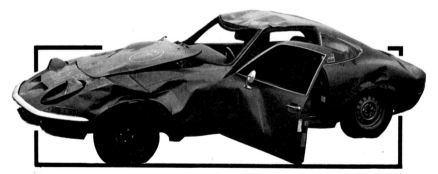

Figure 2.1
Car from which the driver was thrown, showing open door and no compromise of occupant space.

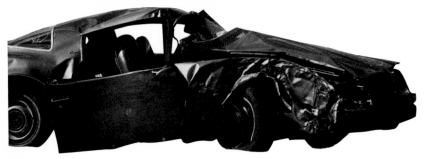

Figure 2.2
Damage to front of car involved in collision with rear of truck. Note rearward displacement of right posterior hood corner and perforation of windshield.

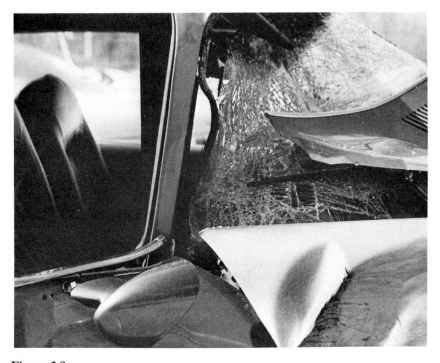

Figure 2.3
Close-up view of right posterior corner of hood that penetrated windshield and inflicted fatal injury to the passenger.

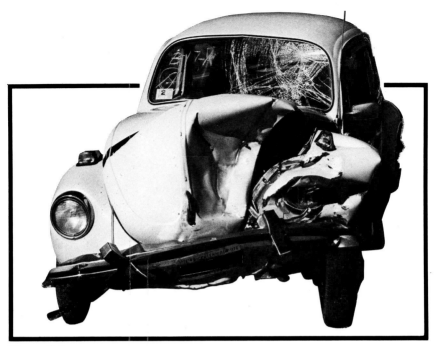

Figure 2.4
Damage to front of Volkswagen involved in front collision.

upper torso restraint would have prevented this injury. This case points out an obvious hazard of this type of hood styling in a forward collision.

Case 3.   A Volkswagon collided with the rear of an automobile that had stopped on the highway. The collision produced considerable damage to the front of the Volkswagon (Fig. 2.4). Considerable rearward displacement of the steering column of the Volkswagon occurred, and the driver decelerated against the steering assembly producing the marked deformation to the steering wheel (Fig. 2.5). The decelerative forces resulting from this collision were of sufficient magnitude to produce a perforating laceration of the right cardiac ventricle. A steering assembly with a greater energy-absorbing capability and the use of an upper-torso and lap-belt restraint system would likely have prevented this fatal injury, even though the crash occurred.[5]

Case 4.   A Ford Torino with an energy-absorbing steering column collided with the left front side of a sedan that had entered the highway from a side road (Fig. 2.6). The driver of the Torino was wearing an upper-torso and lap-belt restraint system; he sustained only a minor facial injury. No compromise of occupant space was noted in the in-

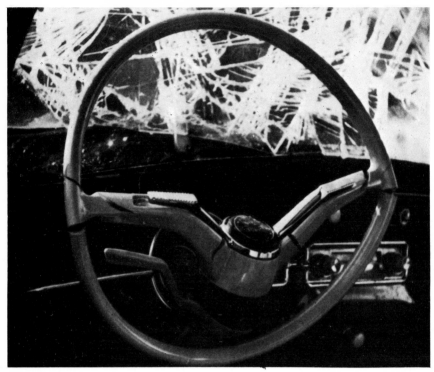

Figure 2.5
Steering wheel of Volkswagen with which driver collided. Notice marked deformation of wheel and rearward displacement of the column.

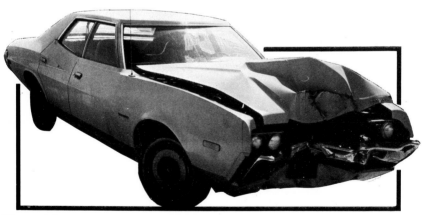

Figure 2.6
Damage to front of Ford Torino in which driver sustained minimal injury.

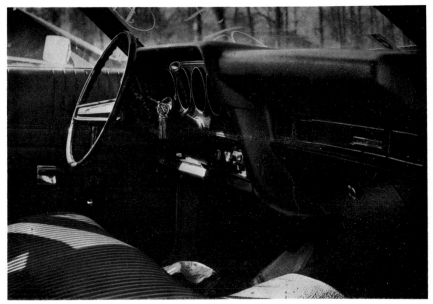

Figure 2.7
Interior of Ford Torino involved in front collision. Notice the adequate occupant space and no deformation of steering wheel or displacement of column. The driver was wearing the upper-torso lap-belt restraint and sustained only minimal injury.

terior of the vehicle, and there was no evidence of rearward displacement or deformation of the steering assembly (Fig. 2.7). Although considerable damage was sustained by the front of the car, the occupant was afforded the benefit of the stopping distance provided by this vehicular crash because he was wearing a restraint system that prevented his coming in contact with the steering assembly. The facial injury probably resulted from his striking his face against the steering wheel as the result of the stretching of the upper-torso belt. This may also have been related to a loosely fastened upper-torso belt.[5]

The tragedy associated with automobile occupant deaths is compounded by the fact that approximately 50% of the fatalities are occurring under potentially survivable conditions. Space available in the occupant area of the vehicle after the crash is vitally important in determining survival, as is the use of the upper-torso and lap-belt restraint systems to prevent ejection and the second collision within the vehicle.[8]

Traditionally, attempts to reduce the morbidity and mortality associated with highway crashes have been directed at accident prevention. To prevent highway accidents from occurring, one must modify the factors contributing to the crashes. These factors include the driver, the vehicle, and the highway. The driver is believed by many to be the cause of most crashes, although one cannot deny the causative role played by defective vehicles and highways in some instances. The difficulty in trying to modify the behavior of more than 100,000,000 drivers limits the effectiveness of accident prevention.

The concept of injury prevention, distinguished from accident prevention, gained in popularity in the 1960s. Injury prevention requires a crashworthy vehicle that provides a safe package for the occupant in the event of a collision. This approach to the highway injury epidemic was aided considerably by the enactment by Congress of Public Law 89–563 in 1966, which authorizes the federal government to promulgate safety standards for automobiles. These standards apply to both operational safety features, such as brakes, lights, and tires, and crash-attenuating features, including energy-absorbing steering assemblies, restraint systems, and door locks.

The chief disadvantage of the belt restraint system is its unpopularity with the public. It is estimated that less than one-third of the occupants of cars use the lap belt, and even fewer persons use the upper-torso and lap-belt combination, which has been a standard item in the front seats of new cars manufactured for sale in the United States since January 1968.

The unpopularity of the belt system has stimulated the development of a passive restraint system, such as the air bag. This passive device inflates rapidly, providing a protective cushion for the car occupant in the event of a front collision. It is activated by a sensor sensitive to a certain magnitude of deceleration. This device is currently installed in some fleet cars on a trial basis to evaluate its performance under true crash conditions. It is hoped that this device or a similar passive device will have wide application in the near future.

Although the lap belt offers definite protection in a crash by preventing ejection and modifying the second collision in the vehicle, it may contribute to injuries in the user. So-called seat-belt injuries have been reported frequently in the medical literature.[4,11,12] The lap belt may be associated with injuries to abdominal viscera, particularly the mesentery, duodenum, and jejunum. A peculiar fracture of the lumbar vertebrae has been described by Smith and Kaufer and is characterized by tension injuries of the lumbar spine.[10] These injuries result in rupture of interspinous ligaments, ligamentum flavum, posterior-longitudinal ligament, and separation of the facet joints. The spinous processes may also be fractured. There may be only minimal evidence of anterior compression of the vertebral bodies. Smith and Kaufer interpret these lesions as the result of a primary tension stress on the lumbar spine as opposed to compression. These lesions usually are not associated with serious neurologic sequelae.

The use of the seat belt by pregnant women in crashes has been associated with fetal death and injury to the uterus; however, there is good reason to believe that without the belt the mother would have been killed. The Committee on Medical Aspects of Automotive Safety of the American Medical Association, after reviewing published studies of nonhuman pregnant primates and studies of pregnant humans in highway crashes, concluded that, in spite of the definite possibility of injuries to the pregnant woman and her fetus resulting from the use of the lap belt in a crash, the overall chances for survival of the mother are much greater if she uses a restraint system, and the three-point belt system is considered superior to the lap belt.[3]

The authors reporting seat-belt injuries emphasize that the occurrence of these injuries is in no way an indictment of the restraint system.[4,10,11] These injuries usually occur in severe crash situations in which fatal injury is the rule. Seat-belt injuries, therefore, are considered acceptable trade-offs for death.

These injury patterns should, however, alert emergency personnel responsible for the care of the crash victim. Knowledge that the victim was wearing a seat belt in a car involved in a front collision should make the physician suspicious of the possibility of intraabdominal or spinal trauma. The physician should be particularly suspicious when there is a belt-induced contusion on the anterior abdominal wall. Hamilton considers such evidence as a sufficient indication for laparotomy.[4]

The motorcycle rider is subjected to greater hazards than the automobile occupant because of inadequate packaging. The number of crashes occurring for 100,000 registered motorcycles shows that fatality from motorcycle crashes is more than twice that for automobile crashes.[2]

PEDESTRIAN ACCIDENTS

The pedestrian presents a special problem because he is more vulnerable to serious injuries than the occupant of an automobile. The pedestrian lacks the packaging afforded by the automobile to its occupant and consequently is the victim of the primary collision. These victims frequently sustain injuries from the initial impact in addition to secondary injuries as the result of striking the ground or some other object often

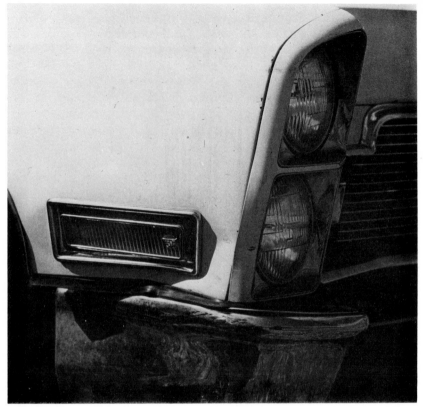

Figure 2.8
Right front edge of automobile that struck pedestrian.

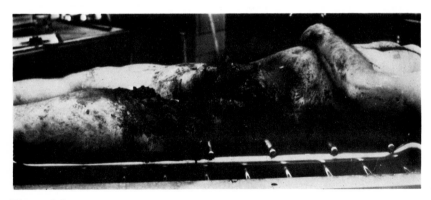

Figure 2.9
Massive injury simulating hemipelvectomy sustained by pedestrian.

a considerable distance from the initial point of contact with the vehicle. The devastating primary injury is demonstrated in case 5.

> Case 5. An adult male was walking along the side of the road when he was struck at hip level by an oncoming automobile with a relatively sharp edge projecting over the head lamp (Fig. 2.8). This contact resulted in the patient's requiring a hemipelvectomy (Fig. 2.9).

There is obvious room for improvement of the front of automobiles, so the impact with pedestrians is better attenuated.

EMERGENCY MEDICAL RESPONSE

These various forms of violence on our roadways provide a major challenge to the emergency medical response system in a community. The small community enjoys no immunity from this challenge; indeed, it may face a greater test of its emergency medical system because of proximity to high-speed interstate expressways as well as recreational areas where snow machines with their attended hazards abound. It is realistic to assume motor vehicle crashes will occur in spite of accident prevention endeavors. As far as the automobile is concerned, the construction of a crashworthy vehicle and the use of restraint systems provide the greatest potential for reduction in morbidity and mortality. Once the injury has occurred, the responsibility is then placed on the emergency response system to effect a salvage of the victims. Most communities have not benefited from the full potential of a sophisticated emergency medical response system. It is hoped that much will be accomplished to correct this deficiency in the next decade.

REFERENCES

[1] Accident Facts. 1973 edition. Chicago, National Safety Council

[2] Committee on Medical Aspects of Automotive Safety: Medical aspects of motorcycle safety. JAMA 204:290–291, 1968

[3] Committee on Medical Aspects of Automotive Safety: Automobile safety belts during pregnancy. JAMA 221:20–21, 1972

[4] Hamilton JB: Seat-belt injuries. Br Med J 4:485–486, 1968

[5] Gikas PW: Mechanisms of injury in automobile crashes. Proceedings of the Congress of Neurological Surgeons. Clin Neurosurg 19:175–190, 1972

[6] Gogler E: Safety devices and safety in vehicle design. Road Accidents. Series Chirurgica. Basle, Switzerland, J.R. Geigy, S.A., 1965, (English translation) pp. 109–137.

[7] Huelke DF, Gikas PW: Ejection—The leading cause of death in automobile accidents. Proceedings of the Tenth Stapp Car Crash Conference. New York, Society of Automotive Engineers, 1966, pp. 156–181

[8] Huelke DF, Gikas PW: Causes of death in automobile accidents. JAMA 203:1100–1107, 1968

[9] Huelke DF, Gikas PW, Hendrix RC: Patterns of injury in fatal automobile accidents. Proceedings of the Sixth Stapp Car Crash Conference. Minneapolis, General Extension Division, University of Minnesota, 1963, pp. 44–58

[10] Smith WS, Kaufer H: Patterns and mechanisms of lumbar injuries associated with lap seat belts. J Bone Joint Surg 51-A:239–254, 1969

[11] Synder RG, Young JW, Snow CC, Hanson P: Seat belt injuries in impact, the prevention of highway injury, ed. ML Selzer, PW Gikas, DF Huelke. Ann Arbor, Highway Safety Research Institute, 1967, pp. 188–210

[12] Taylor FW: Seat-belt injury resulting in regional enteritis and intestinal obstruction. JAMA 215:1154–1155, 1971

William T. Haeck

3

Motor Vehicle Trauma
and Emergency Medical Services

In this chapter the statistics of motor vehicle deaths and trauma will be discussed. The problem was approached in the following sequence: the precrash phase, *i.e.*, effects of highway design, motor vehicle design, driver safety education; the crash phase, *i.e.*, motor vehicle safety requirements; and postcrash phase, *i.e.*, the emergency medical services system. Thought was given to the future trends of motor vehicle death rates.

I am indebted to Roni and Garry Briese and other staff members of the American College of Emergency Physicians for their assistance in preparing this chapter.

27

MOTOR VEHICLE ACCIDENTS

In the light of the available data, the motor vehicle is proving to be one of the major environmental problems of the United States. When one examines the staggering statistics compiled by the National Safety Council in the 1973 edition of *Accident Facts*, it becomes immediately apparent that motor vehicle accidents resulted in 56,600 deaths and 2,100,000 disabling injuries in 1972. The cost of damaged property was $6 billion, and the total cost to our society was a staggering $19.4 billion.[1]

About two of every three motor vehicle deaths in 1972 occurred in places classified as rural. In urban areas, nearly two of five victims were pedestrians; in rural areas, the victims were mostly occupants of motor vehicles. Slightly over half of all deaths occurred in night accidents, the proportion being somewhat higher in urban areas than in rural areas.

Examining the trend in death rates, we find that motor vehicle deaths increased by 3% in 1972 over 1971, while vehicle mileage increased 5%, the number of vehicles increased 4%, and population increased 1%. As a result of the smaller percentage increase in deaths than in vehicle mileage and in registrations, the mileage and registration death rates declined in 1972 from 1971. The population death rate increased. (For the most current statistics, see the most recent issue of *Accident Facts*.) Every 9 min, one motor vehicle death occurs, and every 15 sec someone is injured. If it has taken you a little less than 3 min to read this far, 12 people have been injured in motor vehicle accidents and are, we hope, on the way to a hospital. By the end of today, automobile trauma will have cost our nation another 155 citizens' lives.

Examining the disparity between motor vehicle deaths in urban and rural locations we find that deaths occur more frequently in rural places, but injuries occur more frequently in urban places. Of course, this correlates directly with the fact that more accidents occur in urban areas than in rural areas due to population density and increased traffic. For specific types of accidents, though, the urban/rural proportions vary considerably. For example, only one-third of all deaths occur in urban places, while nearly two-thirds of the pedestrian deaths occur in urban places. Eighty percent of the noncollision deaths happen in rural areas.

Several studies have shown that about one in every four or five patients who die of injury, die of survivable injuries. Waller has stated that in his experience the majority of unnecessary deaths have been the result of two problems—prolonged hypoxia and inadequate blood volume.[7] Both problems are adequately covered in the U.S. Department of Transportation (USDOT) Basic Emergency Medical Technician Training Course.

In most accidents, factors are present relating to the driver, the vehicle, and the road; the interaction of these factors often sets up the series of events that culminate in the mishap. For example, one-half of all accidents occurred when the vehicle skidded after the driver applied brakes, according to data from the Virginia State Police. One-half of all fatal accidents and more than one-half of all injury accidents were caused by this action. Vehicle skidding both before and after the driver applied brakes was reported in more than two-thirds of all accidents.

Drunken Driving

The problem of alcohol use by drivers is also immediately apparent as a major contributing factor in many of the nation's highway deaths. Although the number of drunken driving arrests is up in many parts of the nation owing to an increase in awareness and emphasis on this problem, drunken driving is still being reported by the police in a very substantial share of the accidents.

Drinking is indicated to be a factor in at least half of the fatal motor vehicle accidents, according to special studies. Routine accident reports do not show the same frequency of drinking, but it is believed that such reports understate the frequency, since the necessary time and equipment are not available to perform alcohol tests on all persons involved in accidents.

Due to the continued overrepresentation of alcohol as a contributing factor in traffic crashes, priority must be given to reducing the number of drinking drivers. Since the first problem is that of identifying a drinking driver and then removing him from the road, efforts to accomplish this objective effectively need to be strengthened. Programs to rehabilitate drinking drivers after they are removed from the road are being developed and expanded throughout the nation.

Speed

Excessive speed or speed that is too fast for traffic conditions is another element that has further compounded the fatal crash problem. This factor is involved in about 40% of all traffic crashes, being most prominent in fatalities occurring in the rural areas of the nation where almost 70% of the fatal crashes occur.

Bourke reported in 1965 that speeds below 30 miles per hour accounted for 90% of the accidents, two-thirds of the injuries, and 54%

of the deaths.[3] In another study conducted by Bohlin for the Volvo car manufacturer, 28,000 accident cases were reviewed and the fatalities were found to be spread over the entire speed scale, starting as low as 12 miles per hour.[2]

MOTORCYCLE ACCIDENTS

In 1972, motorcycles, motor scooters, and motorized bicycles, all of which will be referred to as motorcycles, comprised 33.1% of the total vehicle registrations. These vehicles represented 1.2% of the total number of vehicles in all motor vehicle accidents. Therefore, on the basis of the percentage of total vehicles registered, motorcycles have not substantially affected the all-accident picture. These vehicles, however, represented 4.0% of all vehicles involved in fatal accidents. Deaths of operators and passengers of motorcycles totaled 2,700.

Passenger cars have had the opposite experience of two-wheeled motor vehicles. Passenger cars comprised 70.2% of the registered vehicles in 1972. They represented 84.2% of the vehicles involved in all vehicle accidents and 75.3% of those in fatal accidents.

In summary, passenger cars were involved in more than their share of accidents on the basis of vehicle registrations; motorcycles, in less. Passenger cars were involved in less than their share of fatal accidents on the basis of registrations; motorcycles, in more.

Deaths of motorcycle riders increased by 16% in 1972 over 1971. This increase, the fourth in succession, followed 2 years of decreases in motorcycle rider deaths. The exact reason for this is not known, but it has been suggested by some authorities that varying enforcement of helmet laws, changes in the laws, and lack of legislation in some states have an unfavorable effect. The mileage death rate for motorcycle riders in 1972 is estimated at 17 (deaths per 100,000,000 miles of motorcycle travel). The motorcycle mileage death rate of 17 compares with the overall motor vehicle death rate of 4.5, which includes pedestrian and nonoccupant as well as occupant deaths. Collision with another motor vehicle is the predominant type of motorcycle accident. Many people will observe that drivers of the larger vehicles do not always realize that motorcycles, especially motor scooters and motor bicycles, are also motor vehicles and should be treated as such.

PEDESTRIAN ACCIDENTS

Pedestrian deaths have increased to the point at which they account for over half of the traffic fatalities in some large cities and for not less than one-third of the traffic deaths in all urban areas. In the United

States, pedestrian deaths account for one-fifth of all traffic fatalities and between 23% and 38.8% of all road deaths in the less industrialized countries of the world. The pedestrian has the highest mortality of all road users—5.8% compared with 2.4% for vehicle occupants.

Who is the pedestrian victim of automobile accidents? Usually, he falls into one of three categories: the very young, the elderly, or the intoxicated. If he is young, he is likely to be from a poor family. If he is drunk, he is usually a middle-aged male. It is the elderly pedestrian, however, who contributes to the casualty figures far in excess of expectations, both in fatal and nonfatal accidents. His fatal-accident rate starts to climb around age 45, and by age 60, it is nine times that of younger adults.

Huelke and Davis point out that as many pedestrian fatalities happen in crosswalks as outside of them.[6] Pedestrian accidents are more likely to happen at night, in clear weather, under artificial light, and on a dry, straight, asphalt road. The worst month for pedestrian fatalities is December—15% happen then—and the worst time is from 6 P.M. to 9 P.M. A New York study shows that most elderly pedestrians are struck near their home.

What do the traffic experts suggest to lessen the pedestrian accident toll, particularly among the elderly? Some suggestions include (1) longer intervals between stoplight changes at intersections to enable the elderly to cross streets at their speed; (2) more limits on vehicle speeds; (3) gradual relinquishing of driver's control to automated systems; (4) better lighting of roadways in urban areas; (5) traffic engineering and city planning that would make safety of pedestrians a prime concern; and (6) making curbs into inclined planes so that the elderly could negotiate them without stumbling.

DRIVER EDUCATION

Driver education for passenger vehicle operators has as its primary goal a reduction in the number of traffic crashes, injuries, and fatalities that are due to a lack of basic driving knowledge and/or driving skills. Driver education instruction should be provided to all eligible students and the driver education curriculum should be continuously reviewed and upgraded to keep it updated and vigorous. The expanded use of simulation has decreased the cost of driver education by as much as 30%, while maintaining a high level of realistic driving conditions. Computerized multimedia teaching systems in which the computer and student interact with each other are an important supplement to the currently available teaching materials, and they present even more sophisticated teaching programs.

Adult driver education programs need to be expanded and upgraded in the level of instruction by increasing the number of available adult driver education instructors. Consideration should be given to require a basic first aid card as a prerequisite for obtaining a driver's license. Specialized programs should be developed for specialized vehicles such as motorcycles, motor scooters, and snowmobiles. The cost per unit is minimal when compared with the high potential benefits of a sound driver education program.

MOTOR VEHICLE SAFETY REQUIREMENTS

Extensive state-wide motor vehicle inspection and registration procedures should be instituted. The long-range goal is to reduce the incidence of defective vehicles involved in private passenger vehicle crashes by increasing the likelihood that every such vehicle operated on a public highway is properly equipped and maintained in a safe working order. Random checking programs for drivers can include the inspection of drivers' licenses, driver conditions, and vehicle conditions. Since drivers can never be sure when their vehicles will be checked, they are influenced to maintain the good condition of their vehicles.

HIGHWAY SAFETY

Activity in the area of highway safety has significantly increased in the United States since the passage of the Highway Safety Act of 1966. Even though it is encouraging to note that this increased activity has been accompanied by a lowered traffic crash rate, it must be remembered that the amount of damage that continues to be done on our streets and highways is staggering. Although lives lost are irreplaceable, the economic loss associated with the tragic picture is also overwhelming. The traffic crash picture can be improved, and we must continue to utilize every opportunity to reduce the carnage on our highways. A comprehensive, well-planned program for the nation in the area of highway traffic safety is the answer.

The Highway Safety Act of 1966 was passed by the 89th Congress and approved by the President only after a rather searching inquiry by the Senate and the House of Representatives and considerable public discussion of the many important issues involved. To administer this act, the U.S. Department of Transportation and the National Highway Traffic Safety Administration produced the *Highway Safety Program Manual*. This manual contains 16 volumes, which supplement the Highway Safety Program standards and present additional information to assist state and local agencies in implementing their individual highway safety programs. The topics covered in the 16 volumes include motorcycle safety, driver education, driver licensing, alcohol in relation to highway safety, emergency medical services, highway design, pedestrian safety, and police traffic services.

Stimulated by these standards, many states have taken action, such as removing fixed objects within 30 feet of travel lanes of highways. Guardrails have been installed around immovable objects, such as bridges. Breakaway supports are being used for signs and lights. Curves have been grooved to improve tire traction on slippery roads. Freeway medians now have concrete or vegetation barriers to help prevent crossover mishaps. Reflective center markings and stripes at the roadside outline the two-lane highways. On freeways, signs have been improved for readability and placed further from exits to reduce sudden lane crossings. Collisions with fixed objects both on and off freeways accounted for a death total of 4,600. Again we find the discrepancy between the distribution of rural and urban is shown in fixed object collisions in that 2,700 of the total deaths were rural and 1,900 were urban. Improved highway standards, such as those I have already stated, could possibly account for the 1% decrease in collisions with fixed objects from the 1972 figures.

MOTOR VEHICLE SAFETY DESIGN

The recent advances in automobile safety design have taken into account a number of principles employed by professional packing personnel to provide greater protection for fragile items while in transit. The first principle is providing a package that will remain intact and prevent the shipped goods from being thrown out. The package should not collapse under given conditions of force to allow damage to the contents.

The second principle, which is closely related to the first, is providing a structure to shield the inner container. This structure should not be frail, yet it should be capable of resisting force while yielding and absorbing energy applied to it. This function cushions and distributes impact to provide better protection to the inner packing.

The third principle is that the shipped item must be held in one place in an interior package to prevent movement and damage from impact against the inside of the package. The fourth principle states that the inner container, excelsior, styrofoam, or any other means of holding the item inside the shipping container must be capable of transmitting forces to the strongest part of the item.

These principles have been applied to automobile design. The application of one principle without the remaining three can defeat the purpose of the single principle provided. Examples of this work include collapsible steering columns, padded interior design, high seat backs, seat belts, pin-locking doors, steel reinforced doors and roofs, a downward deflecting engine, and removal of objects protruding into the interior of the car.

Vehicle design is a continuous series of engineering compromises, and the inclusion of one factor or group of factors to eliminate one problem may well create a series of new problems. We know that the possibility of crashes cannot be removed totally from any transportation system. Whatever mode of travel we choose, it possesses certain inherent dangers and risks to the user and, unfortunately, since we cannot remain immobile, these risks must be taken. Yet, current technology has brought us a long way toward eliminating a major portion of the hazards in our transportation systems.

In the highway transportation area, many innovative concepts once applied have contributed a great deal toward eliminating or reducing the severity of traffic crashes. Almost everybody has some conception of how seat belts contribute to personal safety. People know that belts reduce injuries caused by striking "hostile" surfaces in the car interior. This is the so-called second collision. The first collision occurs when the vehicle strikes or is struck by another object. The second collision occurs when the occupant of the vehicle is flung against the instrument panel, windshield, windows, side panels, roof, doorknobs, steering wheel, etc. Any one occupant can have several second collisions during a single accident depending on how much he gets tossed around the car. People are also aware that belts increase safety by holding the occupant inside the car, avoiding injury from ejection.

People are generally less aware of other contributions. For example, in a collision, the occupants can fly into or roll over each other; by keeping their seat belts in place, the chance of the occupants' becoming another source of injury to each other is reduced. Belts can also help prevent accidents. By keeping the driver firmly in place, they increase his control of the vehicle. By keeping the driver in a comfortable position, they can reduce fatigue and make driving a little safer. Children who are firmly buckled in are less likely to distract the driver's attention from the problems of driving.

However, the average person's knowledge in this area is probably superficial and somewhat vague. Maybe that is one reason why belt usage is so low; people "sort of know" that belts help, but they do not know exactly what they do or how well they do it. Again we are faced with the problem of public education. The nonuser should be bombarded from all sides with a well-coordinated campaign for seat-belt utilization.

Some safety campaigns set impossible, unattainable goals. It is useless to tell somebody to drive safely, and the public knows it. You can tell people to drive carefully until you are blue in the face, but there will still be accidents. Actually, don't most drivers really believe that they already drive carefully? But when you tell people to "buckle up" you are recommending a specific action that is completely within the realm of possibility. All messages should aim toward achieving a definite observable, measurable behavior, as opposed to attitude-illiciting messages.

During the actual crash the passenger in a recently manufactured automobile is protected from injury by a number of devices and concepts. We see increasing use of seat belts, the air bag, the integration of collapsible steering columns, pin-locking doors, and laminated safety glass windows. Recent windshield advances have shown that glass with controlled deformation characteristics (the ability to yield and stretch under moderate impact and the ability to yield and deform without the plastic lamina tearing under severe impact) have brought about a reduction in the severity of lacerative injuries to the face, head, and neck.

An item that is extremely dangerous to human life in a crash deceleration is the older steering-wheel assemblies of passenger cars. Steering-wheel assemblies include the steering wheel, hub, column, horn ring, steering control blocks, and placement of same. In crash decelerations, a large number of older steering-wheel designs allowed high-impact loads to be transferred to the driver's chest and head. Cast horn rings and trim found in early models fractured and exposed sharp unyielding edges that produced lacerations and head damage. Energy-absorbing steering columns have reduced the incidence of injuries of this type seen in emergency departments.

The improvements in automobile design, automobile safety standards, highway design, and other ancillary areas are apparent. But, we will never be able to stop all motor vehicle accidents. When the accident has happened, the emergency medical services system begins to function.

EMERGENCY MEDICAL SERVICES SYSTEM

What is an emergency medical services system? It is best defined by taking a good look at the basic sequence of events that an acutely ill or injured patient will need to go through to return him to society as a full functional person. There are six basic components to the emergency medical services system. (1) Discovery and notification: Somebody must find the victim and call for help. (2) Dispatch of help: Whatever agency, public or private, receives the call for help, must quickly dispatch the appropriate vehicles and individuals to help the victim. (3) Onsite care: The individual or individuals who discover the victim must begin effective care for the victim and turn that care over to better-trained individuals when they arrive. This care must continue until the victim reaches the emergency care facility. (4) Transportation: The victim must be moved from the point of discovery to a facility where definitive care can be administered. (5) Initial care in the facility: Life-threatening conditions must be corrected, the victim stabilized, and a diagnosis made so that he may receive definitive care. (6) Definitive care: The care that will eventually return him to society.

It is appalling to realize that in many places in the United States, if someone is in an accident or is critically ill, he may wait at least an hour for an ambulance, and, even worse, he needs to be conscious and have some medical knowledge to instruct the ambulance attendants on caring for him, so he can have a safe trip to the hospital.

Although a system may be lacking in a community, there is not one community that is devoid of the essential building blocks for the development of such a system. The manpower is available but often untrained. The transportation and communication elements exist, but the basic plans for the development of an integrated system are frequently lacking.

Inherent in this lack of organization comes the absence of agency cooperation and coordination and the evaluation of programs. Without this organization and coordination, it is impossible to know whether the needs for the improvement of the delivery of emergency medical services for a community are due to a lack of manpower, training, equipment, vehicles, communications, or other factors.

Coexisting with these weaknesses is the fragmentation of programs and funding for emergency medical services at the state level. Since all emergency medical services are, in fact, a subsystem of the total health care system, there is a need to provide continuity of care through all components of the emergency medical services system.

A break anywhere along the chain of an emergency medical services system will cause grave socioeconomic losses to the country; a loss that can only in part be estimated in dollars and cents.

To better understand the emergency medical services system, I have introduced a flow chart (Fig. 3.1) that concentrates on heightening the elements and decision points in sequence. The decision points will tend to fall at the "boundaries," *e.g.,* consumer/emergency medical treatment—emergency medical treatment/transport—transport/hospital.

The elements of the flow chart may be described in terms of their number, distribution, and operational capacity. There also are subsystem boundaries, *i.e.,* hospital catchment areas, operating zones of vehicles, aircraft, etc., and competency limits of personnel. Their interactions may be described in terms of rules of procedure relating to the use of the elements across boundaries (dispatch rules, emergency department procedures, radio consultation rules, etc.).

Incident Occurs; Incident Detected; Call for Assistance

The number 911 has been accepted by the American Telephone and Telegraph Company as the national, three-digit, emergency number. Having a number such as this avoids the confusion of multiple telephone listings and jurisdictional disputes. It allows for rapid response to calls for service for the public and for the efficient utilization of manpower resulting from the consolidation of dispatching services. It also will eliminate duplication of effort; in any busy urban area it is rather common to have an emergency reported to more than one police or fire department, resulting in the response by more units than are required by the situation. This central communications center eliminates this problem with a considerable savings to the taxpayer.

The true value of a single emergency telephone number service in any community is in improving the citizen's ability to obtain emergency assistance. The ultimate burden and responsibility for implementing the 911 emergency number lies with local governments. It is here that the decision must be made, the costs incurred, and the problems resolved.

Dispatch Receives the Call; Ambulance Notified; Other Related Agencies Notified

A central emergency resource management center is essential to the proper organization of emergency medical services resources and follows as a corollary to the centralized, single notification number. Regardless of the extent of the services offered by this resource management center, or the organizational structure, such a center effectively becomes the known entry point into the emergency medical services system, and a place where persons are knowledgeable of the resources and routing procedures necessary to have a proper response made to the call for assistance. This is the system element that links all the other system elements together through telecommunications.

Arrive on the Scene; Emergency Medical Procedures Instituted

The most serious problem now facing emergency medical services in the United States is the lack of education and training of ambulance

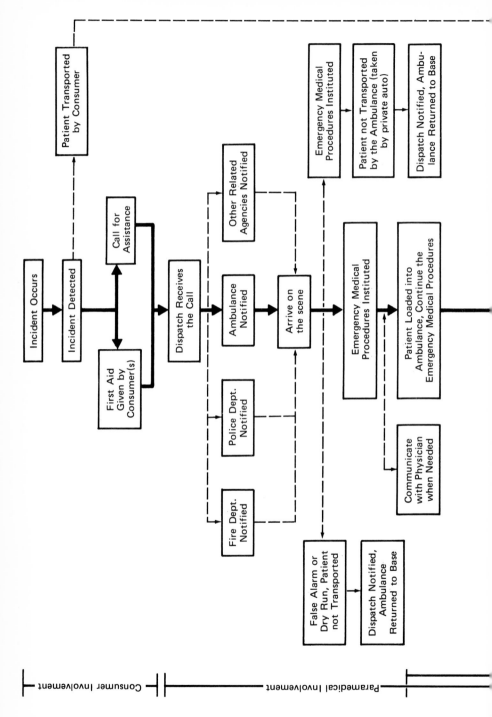

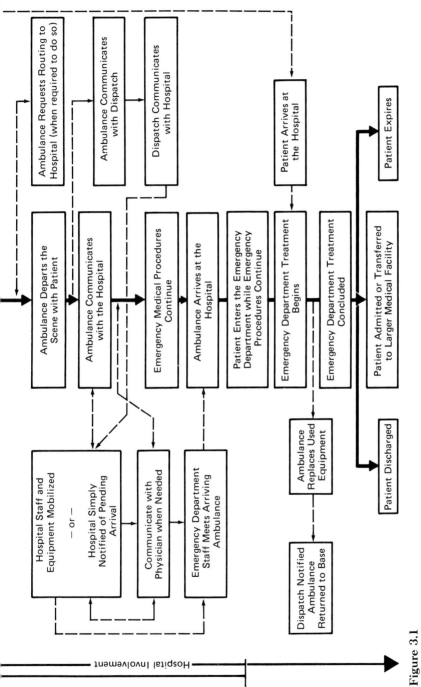

Figure 3.1
Emergency medical services flow chart.

personnel. The growing importance of emergency medical services justifies a professional status comparable to that of other existing technical medical services. Individuals who qualify for this vocation through standard national certification should be known as emergency medical technicians (EMT).

The levels of proficiency to be attained by the USDOT basic emergency medical technician training course (81 hours) are goals that can be reached in most areas of the country within a reasonable time.

Although the greatest potential for the saving of life and reduction of preventable disability is at the scene of accidental injury or life-threatening illness, this potential will not be realized until ambulance personnel are qualified to carry out measures now applied by lay assistants in emergency departments or by medical corpsmen in combat areas.

To attain this goal, accredited hospital and community college training programs must be established that will produce professional emergency medical technicians and emergency department assistants. The ambulance attendant must be fully engaged in emergency care in an established career pattern that provides attractive compensation, prestige, and recognition deserving of his services as a member of the emergency care team.

Some "traditional" discrepencies in emergency medical technician training include little situational-practical exercises, a lack of psychological emotional training (both for the EMT and for his patient), and a near absence of automobile extrication training. As training needs such as these become more obvious, they are being integrated into the more progressive EMT courses.

Patient Loaded; Ambulance Departs; Ambulance Communicates with Hospital

No longer is it necessary to conduct "demonstration projects" on the effectiveness of on-the-scene emergency medical care and adequate emergency medical transportation. The fact is that, in communities all around the United States, lives are being saved through the use of both basic and advanced emergency medical technicians. Examples of such cities are well known. The outstanding results that have been achieved in these cities would not be possible without a commitment from their political leaders for expenditures of monies for new ambulances, supportive equipment, and excellent training.

This training, along with the establishment of the National Registry of Emergency Medical Technicians, is leading to standardization of EMT ratings and to the needed degree of professionalization. Wherever such training programs have been in effect, physicians in hospital emergency departments have seen immediate improvements in the quality of care provided prior to the patients' arrival in the emergency department.

Ambulance Arrives at the Hospital;
Emergency Department Treatment Begins

Prehospital patient care should merge almost imperceptably with that continued in the emergency department, and this chain of emergency care must have continuity if the patient is to receive the greatest benefit. Excellent patient care is our first responsibility.

The training of the emergency medical technician is most appropriately conducted by the emergency physician because he should be most informed about the emergency medical services in his community. He can more easily be considered expert in the field than any other professional. The improvements in quality of care the emergency physician generates will therefore directly relate to the chosen goals of his career. The emergency department of today reflects the necessary innovation to furnish prompt primary care to patients of all ages with all kinds of emergency health problems.

Emergency Department Treatment Concluded;
Patient Admitted, Transferred, or Discharged

We have learned that specialty areas of the hospital, such as coronary care units, intensive care units, respiratory care units, burn centers, and trauma centers, can save lives that were formerly lost. The many advances and special procedures [central venous pressure (CVP), heart pacing, open heart surgery, artificial kidneys] are all relatively recent developments to save lives on demand.

We all are aware, however, that not all hospitals can support these facilities. We will have to consolidate and specialize and categorize our hospital facilities to get the most effective emergency health care for each dollar spent. Regional planning is essential.

FUTURE CONSIDERATIONS

Most certainly the recent advances in federal vehicle safety standards, state and federal highway legislation, emergency medical telecommunications, and emergency medical training are only a preview of things to come.

The passage of the Emergency Medical Services Systems Act of 1973 has redirected federal efforts in this vital area. More and more states have adopted comprehensive emergency medical services legislation requiring upgraded training and up-to-date ambulances.

> What relationship will the energy shortage have to motor vehicle deaths? Reductions in deaths during the 1973 Thanksgiving holiday and 1973 Christmas holiday compared with these same periods in 1972 have already been widely quoted in the press as an indication that the energy shortage has already begun to reduce motor vehicle deaths. Such conclusions are premature.
> There is considerable evidence, if all other aspects of the situation were unchanging, the decreasing size of the cars in the vehicle population would tend to generate more severe and more frequent losses.[4]

In a two-vehicle accident the small car is more likely to collide with a larger car simply because there are more large cars on the road. When this small car collides with the larger car, the small car and its passengers generally get the worst of the bargain. Much of the problem stems from the mix of five sizes of cars—subcompact, compact, intermediate, standard, and luxury—from under 1 ton to 2.5 tons. The general rule is that the larger the car, the more protection its occupants have.

A Transportation-Department-sponsored study of accidents involving 420,000 cars in New York state in 1968 showed that 3.1% of the people involved in crashes of big cars weighing an average of 4,800 lb. were killed or seriously injured. But the rate of death or serious injury rose to 4% in intermediate cars averaging 3,700 lb., to 6.4% in domestic compact cars averaging 2,800 lb., and 9.6% in foreign compacts averaging 1,900 lb.

Another point to consider is the reduction in speed from the previously average top speed of 70 miles per hour to present maximum speed of 55 miles per hour.

> Available data suggests that if all other aspects were unchanging, it is likely that reduced speeds would result in fewer deaths and injuries, but little appreciable change in crash frequencies. Also, decreased travel speeds result in increased travel times, and this will increase traffic density. The effect of this increase in "time exposure" is unknown.
> Passenger car mileage may decrease, and it is likely that substantial decreases in vehicle mileage would result in some reductions in highway losses. It is not possible at this time, however, to scientifically predict what, if any, these reductions would be.
> Vehicle occupancy rates may increase, meaning that the chances of

injury in any crash are increased. In addition, it is probable that increased occupancy rates in small cars adversely affect the braking and handling characteristics to a much greater extent than do increased occupancy rates in large cars. Therefore, the combination of small cars and higher occupancy rates would possibly tend to increase crash frequencies.

The average age of vehicles in use may increase if people disproportionately use older vehicles because of their better gasoline consumption. The effect of a change in the average age of vehicles in use is uncertain, although many of the older vehicles would not be designed to satisfy the more recent federal vehicle safety standards.

The extent and duration of the energy shortage is not predictable, although there is apparently no doubt that there will continue to be at least short-term shortages of gasoline and truck fuels. In view of the uncertain short-term prospects and the many aspects of the new situation that are changing, it is not possible to predict with any confidence what the short-term effects, even as to direction, will be on each of the various categories of highway losses.[5]

CONCLUSION

The American medical community during the past decade has become increasingly aware of the problems resulting from today's highly mechanized and mobile society. In 1972, motor vehicle accidents resulted in 56,600 deaths and 2,100,000 disabling injuries, at a total cost to our society of $19.4 billion.

An effective emergency medical services system throughout the nation will assist substantially in the reduction of motor vehicle mortality and morbidity.

REFERENCES

[1] Accident Facts. 1973 edition. Chicago, National Safety Council

[2] Bohlin Nl: Proceedings of the Eleventh Stapp Car Crash Conference. Warrendale, Pa., Society of Automotive Engineers, 1967, pp. 299–308

[3] Bourke CJ: Efficacy of car safety belts. J Ir Med Assn 57:110–117, 1965

[4] Highway Loss Reduction Status Report. Insurance Institute for Highway Safety 8 (Dec. 20, 1973)

[5] Ibid.

[6] Huelke DF, Davis RA: Proceedings of a Conference on the Prevention of Highway Injury. Ann Arbor, University of Michigan, Highway Safety Research Institute, 1967

[7] Waller JA: Urban oriented methods, failure to solve rural emergency care problems. JAMA 266:1441–1446, 1973

SUGGESTED READING

Accidental death and disability: The neglected disease of modern society. Washington, Division of Medical Sciences, National Academy of Sciences, National Research Council. Reprinted by the U.S. Department of Health, Education, and Welfare, 1966

Accident Facts. 1973 edition. Chicago, National Safety Council

A guide for a workshop to identify improving emergency medical services in the community. East Lansing, Mich., American College of Emergency Physicians, 1972

Emergency department management guide. East Lansing, Mich., American College of Emergency Physicians, Committee on Hospitals, 1971

Are small cars safe? Changing Times, The Kiplinger Magazine, October 1973, pp. 11–13

Bacon, Selklen, Daskam: Studies of driving and drinking. Brunswick, N.J., Center of Alcohol Studies, Rutgers University, 1968

Briese G, Peeler B et al: A ten-year plan for an emergency medical services system—Florida. Jacksonville, Florida Division of Health, 1972

Carraro B: A look at motorcycle accidents in 1972. Traffic Safety, December, 1973

Developing emergency medical services guidelines for community councils. Chicago, American Medical Association Commission on Emergency Medical Services, 1970

Eclitor DA: The role of the drinking driver in traffic accidents. Indianapolis, Department of Police Administration, Indiana University, 1964

Emergency Medical Services Act of 1972. Hearings before the Subcommittee on Public Health and Environment of the Committee on Interstate and Foreign Commerce, House of Representatives. Washington, U.S. Government Printing Office, 1972

Emergency Medical Services. Proceedings of the First Regional Conference. Atlanta, May, 1972

Emergency medical services—Recommendations for an approach to an urgent national problem. Proceedings of the Airlie Conference on Emergency Medical Services, Warrenton, Va., May, 1967

Emergency Medical Services Systems Development Act of 1973. Hearings before the Subcommittee on Health of the Committee on Labor and Public Welfare, U.S. Senate. Washington, U.S. Government Printing Office, 1973

Essential equipment for ambulances. Chicago, Bull Coll Surg, 1970, pp. 7–13

Horton JR (ed): Ambulance service journal articles. New York, Medical Examination Publishing Co., Inc., 1971

Model program? How California cut road deaths. U.S. News and World Report, May 8, 1972, p. 102

911—A summary report. Washington, National Service to Regional Councils, 1970

Organization for Economic Cooperation and Development: Lighting, visibility, and accidents, Paris, 1971

The critically injured patient concept and the Illinois statewide plan for trauma

centers. Springfiled, Illinois Department of Public Health, 1971
Waters JM et al: The effect of a modern emergency medical care system in reducing automobile crash deaths. J Trauma 13:645–647, 1973
White RD: Physician's role in ambulance service. JACEP 1(6): 39–42, 1972

A. James Lewis

4

The Cardiac Patient

The leading cause of death in the United States is coronary artery disease, accounting for approximately 600,000 deaths per year.[32] This chapter will deal with the emergency management of the cardiac patient, and address itself to the prevention and management of sudden death due to coronary artery disease.

SUDDEN CARDIAC DEATH

Definition

The term *sudden death* has been variously defined. An international committee sponsored by the Scientific Council on Atherosclerosis and

Ischemic Heart Disease of the International Society of Cardiology and by the Councils on Atherosclerosis and Epidemiology of the American Heart Association has recommended the following definition: "Sudden unexpected (natural) death is defined as death occurring instantaneously or within an estimated 24 hours of the onset of acute symptoms or signs."[27]

Epidemiology

In a study of sudden death in Baltimore, Maryland, Kuller found that 60% of all deaths due to coronary disease occurred outside the hospital within 24 hours of symptom onset.[15] Other investigators have reported that 40–75% of all deaths from acute myocardial infarction (AMI) occur during the first hour; 60–90% occur within 24 hours.[8] Bondurant estimated that 125,000 persons per year under age 65 die prior to hospitalization from coronary artery disease.[1] Hence, the greatest mortality from coronary artery disease occurs prior to hospitalization and within 24 hours of the onset of AMI.

Relationship of Arrhythmias to Sudden Cardiac Death

Experience in the coronary care unit (CCU) has shown that the most common cause of sudden cardiac death is ventricular fibrillation (VF).[21] When primary (that is, unassociated with left ventricular failure or cardiogenic shock), normal cardiac rhythm can usually be restored by prompt defibrillation. The occurrence of primary VF when promptly treated should not adversely affect the prognosis of the patient with AMI.[21] Ventricular fibrillation is often preceded by premature ventricular contractions (PVC) and if controlled by suppressive antiarrhythmic therapy, the incidence of VF may be reduced.[20,21,33] The application of these principles in the CCU has resulted in a decline in the hospital mortality of AMI from 30–40% to 17–20%.[14] There has been, however, only a 2–3% decline in total mortality, since death occurs prior to hospitalization in the majority of patients.[20]

Studies in which patients have been monitored electrocardiographically during the early hours following the onset of AMI have confirmed the high incidence of VF during the initial hours following symptom onset. Pantridge and Geddes found the risk of VF to be 15 times greater during the first 4 hours than during the remainder of the initial 12 hours.[26] Lawrie found that 38 of 71 patients (54%) developed VF during the initial 4 hours, and 50 (70%) developed this arrhythmia within 12 hours.[16]

Lewis and associates noted a significant incidence of major ar-

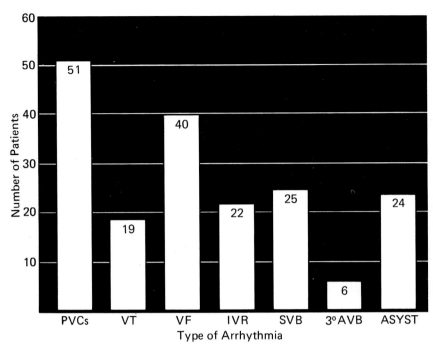

Figure 4.1
Prehospital incidence of arrhythmias in 162 cardiac patients. Multiple arrhythmias frequently occurred in a single patient. Premature ventricular contractions (PVCs); ventricular tachycardia (VT); ventricular fibrillation (VF); idi-
oventricular rhythm (IVR); supraventricular bradycardia (SVB); third-degree
atrioventricular block (3° AVB); ventricular asystole (ASYST).

rhythmias in 162 cardiac patients monitored in a mobile intensive care
unit (MICU) prior to hospitalization (Fig. 4.1).[17] Of special concern was
the occurrence of PVC in 51 (31.4%) and VF in 40 (24.5%).

Pantridge has noted the high incidence of bradyarrhythmias during
the early phase of AMI and has stressed their importance in the genesis
of sudden death. He noted that 32% of patients with acute inferior MI
developed a supraventricular bradyarrhythmia during the first hour
after symptom onset.[25]

PREVENTION OF SUDDEN CARDIAC DEATH

The major emphasis in the reduction of sudden cardiac death must be
placed on the early institution of antiarrhythmic therapy prior to the

time the patient reaches the CCU. This is a complex task, the essential features of which are discussed further.

Identification of the Population at Risk

Although it is not possible to delineate all persons at risk for sudden cardiac death, a significant number can be identified. In the Tecumseh study, 45 of 98 deaths from coronary artery disease were sudden.[3] It was found that the incidence of sudden death was 15-fold or greater among persons with either symptomatic coronary artery disease, diabetes mellitus, or hypertensive heart disease. Two or more of these risk factors were found in 51% of those who died suddenly.

The Framingham study has suggested that sudden death is more common in the obese, particularly when associated with hypercholesterolemia, hypertension, or diabetes.[13] The Framingham study also implicated heavy cigarette smoking with sudden death.[12] Eighty-four percent of the sudden death group in the Tecumseh study had a prior electrocardiographic (ECG) abnormality. Of particular importance were the presence of ventricular conduction abnormalities (right bundle branch block with left anterior hemiblock, and isolated left bundle branch block), evidence of previous myocardial infarction, left ventricular hypertrophy, and PVCs. In an earlier report, Chiang and associates[4] found that 10 of 165 persons over age 30 with PVCs died suddenly, compared with 35 of 3,459 persons without this arrhythmia ($p < 0.01$).

Professional Education

Efforts to make the physician better able to cope with the problem of AMI and sudden death should stress the following areas.[33]

Familiarization with the early signs and symptoms of AMI and the unstable anginal syndromes. Although sudden death may occur without warning, recognizable prodromal symptoms are often present. In a study of 100 patients with AMI, Solomon and associates found that 65 experienced prodromal symptoms during a 2-month period prior to the MI.[30] Chest pain was present in 59. Kuller found that 23% of persons who died suddenly of atherosclerotic heart disease had been seen by a physician during the week before death.[15]

Certain clinical syndromes (the so-called preinfarction, unstable angina, or intermediate syndromes) deserve special mention since they signal the potential for imminent AMI or sudden death.[9] In brief, these include (1) angina of recent onset, often with ordinary or less than ordinary activity; (2) crescendo angina, a marked increase in frequency or severity of a previously stable anginal syndrome; (3) angina with minimal exertion or at rest; (4) Prinzmetal's angina—a variant form of ischemic chest pain unassociated with exertion and characterized by ST segment elevation on the ECG during the pain.[28]

Suspicion of AMI or of an unstable anginal syndrome is a definite indication for the immediate institution of continuous ECG surveillance and appropriate antiarrhythmic therapy. Life-threatening arrhythmias, such as VF, can occur during the course of an unstable anginal syndrome, and, if promptly treated, AMI does not necessarily result.

Although it is not widely appreciated, a normal appearing ECG does not exclude AMI in its early stages. This factor is well illustrated in Figure 4.2. A normal ECG should never be the basis for reassuring a patient who has experienced an episode of prolonged chest pain that "nothing is wrong."

Competence in basic life support (cardiopulmonary resuscitation) and advanced life support (the recognition and management of life-threatening arrhythmias). Physicians who are responsible for patient management should be required to undergo training in basic life support and to demonstrate competence on a yearly basis. Such a requirement would be an appropriate condition for hospital staff membership. In addition, those physicians who practice in a hospital emergency department or intensive care unit should be capable of recognizing life-threatening arrhythmia and defibrillation and providing appropriate drug therapy and airway management.

Familiarization with emergency facilities within the community. The physician must become aware of what is available for prehospital emergency care (*e.g.*, a paramedic-manned mobile intensive care unit) and the capabilities of the various hospital emergency departments. The physician would not be able to advise his patients properly without this information.

Public Education

In a prospective study of 134 patients with AMI, Moss and Goldstein found that the average time between the onset of symptoms and the decision to call for medical assistance was 3 hours.[22] It has already been noted that the highest mortality from AMI occurs during the initial hours following symptom onset.[8,15,16,26] The importance of organized

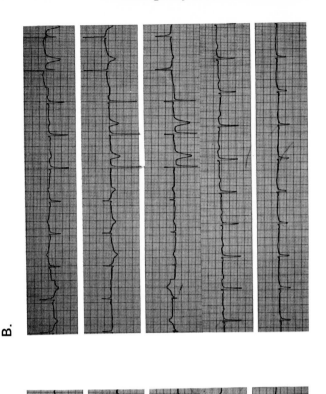

Figure 4.2
ECG of a 50-year-old man with chest pain of 2 hours duration. **A.** ECG taken in emergency department and revealing only nonspecific changes. **B.** Within 24 hours deep T-wave inversion had occurred. These changes persisted and were accompanied by enzyme elevation. The diagnosis of acute subendocardial infarction was made.

programs of public education, such as those sponsored by the American Heart Association and its affiliates, cannot be overemphasized.

Such programs should stress (1) familiarization with the warning symptoms and signs of AMI; (2) the necessity to seek medical assistance promptly; (3) development of a plan of action to obtain medical assistance by the most expeditious means, including summoning a mobile intensive (or coronary) care unit, summoning an ordinary ambulance or rescue squad, going directly to the hospital emergency department by private automobile, or calling a private physician; and (4) instruction in basic life-support techniques (cardiopulmonary resuscitation) for the relatives and associates of known high-risk patients.

This instruction is necessary because of the high incidence of cardiac arrest outside the hospital and the finite period of time necessary for trained rescue personnel to arrive. This concept has been endorsed by the American Heart Association.[31]

Development of a System for Delivery of Prehospital Coronary Care

Entry into the system. A fundamental concept in any emergency medical system is that the consumer must first recognize the need for emergency medical service. He then must know what type of emergency service is available, *e.g.*, fire department rescue squad, commercial ambulance, etc. Finally, there must be a readily available method of obtaining the emergency service. In most communities this involves a telephone call to a physician, the police department, the fire department, an ambulance company, or the telephone operator. Within Los Angeles County, for example, there are 54 separate telephone numbers for emergency medical service. The implementation of the universal emergency telephone number (911) would greatly reduce or eliminate the confusion that the public must feel when confronted by an unexpected medical emergency.

Development of mobile life-support units. A major advancement in emergency medical care in recent years has been the development of mobile life-support units (LSUs). Such units are designed to institute definitive forms of therapy in life-threatening situations before the patient reaches the hospital. The impetus to the development of such units in the United States was the demonstration by Pantridge and associates in 1966 of the value of antiarrhythmic therapy in AMI prior to hospitalization.[26]

The mobile coronary care unit. Initially, such mobile LSUs were reserved exclusively for the heart attack patient[11,19,26] and, hence, necessitated the development of new and often expensive rescue services parallel to already existing emergency facilities. The early mobile coronary care units (MCCUs) were staffed by physicians and/or nurses; paramedics are now utilized on some.

The mobile intensive care unit. A different approach that involved the upgrading of already existing rescue resources was adopted by Nagel in 1969.[24] In addition to training the members of the Miami Fire Department Rescue Service in cardiopulmonary resuscitation, each rescue unit was equipped with a portable radiotransceiver for transmission of voice and ECG to the hospital and with a defibrillator.

Following the example of Nagel in the use of paramedical personnel to administer more definitive forms of therapy outside the hospital, Lewis and associates developed a pilot program in Los Angeles County in 1969.[17] The purpose of this program was to enhance the capabilities of already existing emergency rescue personnel and resources, permitting the institution of definitive therapy for a wide spectrum of emergencies prior to hospitalization. This resulted in the formation of a multipurpose MICU manned by highly trained paramedics. Similar systems were developed by both Cobb[5] and Rose.[29]

The following discussion will be based on the mobile intensive care program within Los Angeles County because of the author's familiarity with it.

Training of MICU paramedics. Since emergency medical care within Los Angeles County and its many municipalities is a responsibility of the fire departments, fire fighters experienced in rescue work were selected for special paramedic training. The training program has undergone considerable expansion since its development in 1969. The curriculum now consists of a 20-week course.[17] This is comparable in content to the Emergency Medical Technician II course developed by the Department of Health, Education, and Welfare.

During the initial or didactic phase, the paramedic trainee spends 8 weeks of intensive study covering basic medical terminology, anatomy, physiology, and the diagnosis and treatment of a wide variety of medical and surgical conditions. An important aspect of this phase involves the interpretation of cardiac arrhythmias and the use of cardiovascular drugs. The student also receives instruction in special techniques, such as venipuncture, nasogastric intubation, and pulmonary ventilation.

The second phase of training, lasting 12 weeks, involves clinical experience. During the first 4 weeks, the trainee is assigned to the hospital emergency room and intensive care units where he is taught by demonstration and performance how to obtain the essential features of a medical history and how to perform a limited physical examination. Under supervision he is permitted to handle a variety of medical and surgical emergency situations. He responds with the hospital cardiac arrest team and performs closed chest cardiac massage, pulmonary ventilation, and defibrillation. He is supervised in the administration of drugs by the intravenous and intracardiac routes. Additional training in the hospital includes mastering the technique of venipuncture and learning the fundamentals of emergency childbirth.

During the final 8 weeks of clinical experience, the student is assigned to an MICU. During this time, he gains valuable field experience on actual emergency runs under the close supervision of experienced paramedics.

During each stage of his training, the paramedic must pass both oral and written examinations. In addition to successfully passing these examinations, he must demonstrate the ability to apply this knowledge under field conditions.

As of December 1973, 367 paramedics had been trained and certified under the auspices of the Los Angeles County Paramedic Program. Forty-seven MICUs are now in operation in association with 19 base station hospitals. Although most trainees have been fire fighters, selected civilian ambulance attendants have also received paramedic training. Plans have been formulated to incorporate the civilian ambulance companies into this program.

MICU operation.   A typical paramedic team, consisting of two trained paramedics, is assigned to an MICU based at strategically located fire

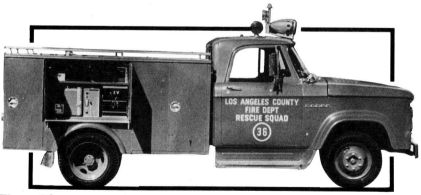

Figure 4.3
Utility truck with MICU equipment (stored in side panel), in addition to fire fighting and extrication gear.

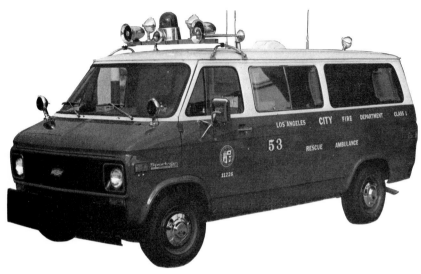

Figure 4.4
Rescue ambulance used by the Los Angeles City Fire Department paramedics.

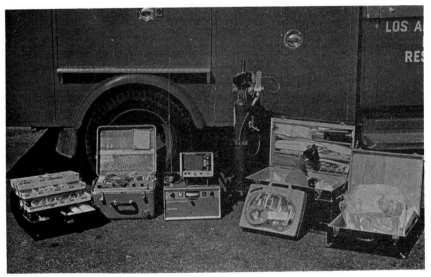

Figure 4.5
Portable MICU equipment used by all paramedic teams in the Los Angeles program. Shown from left to right: drug box; radiotransceiver (battery powered); defibrillator and oscilloscope (battery powered); oxygen; suction unit; box containing intravenous solutions, splints, bandages, and other miscellaneous equipment; and an obstetric kit.

stations. The type of vehicle used varies among the several fire departments. The principal rescue vehicle of the Los Angeles County Fire Department is a utility truck with no patient-transport capability (Fig. 4.3). The paramedic teams of the Los Angeles City Fire Department and of several of the smaller municipalities within Los Angeles County use conventional ambulances (Fig. 4.4). Each rescue unit is equipped with a portable radio transceiver, defibrillator, oscilloscope, ventilatory and suction apparatus, emergency childbirth kit, intravenous solutions, and selected drugs. Conventional rescue equipment is also available (Fig. 4.5). This equipment is portable and can be brought directly to the patient, rather than moving the patient into the rescue vehicle.

When a call for assistance is received by the fire department, the appropriate MICU is dispatched. Upon arrival at the emergency scene, pertinent historical information and vital signs are obtained. If emergency therapy, such as cardiac massage and pulmonary ventilation, is necessary, it is immediately started. When appropriate, ECG electrodes are attached and the ECG rhythm is displayed on the oscilloscope. If VF is present, countershock is immediately applied. The paramedic then contacts the hospital base station by radio, where a physician or specially certified registered nurse directs further therapy (Fig. 4.6).

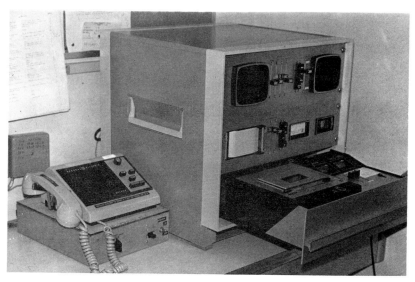

Figure 4.6
Hospital base station. Transceiver (left). Console containing an ECG demodulator, ECG oscilloscope, strip chart recorder, and a cassette tape recorder used to make permanent records of all ECG and voice transmissions (right).

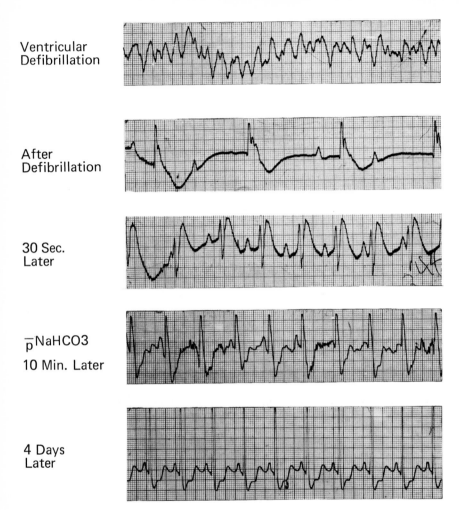

Figure 4.7
ECGs of a 62-year-old man with VF due to AMI.

The physician (or nurse) is advised of the patient's history and vital signs. The ECG can then be transmitted. The paramedics may be instructed to start an intravenous solution and to administer appropriate drugs, such as lidocaine, when PVCs are noted. When a life-threatening situation is present, every effort is made to stabilize the patient's condition before transport to the hospital. If these efforts have been successful, a high-speed ambulance ride with red light and siren can be avoided.

Figure 4.7 shows the resuscitation of a 62-year-old man with VF due to AMI. The ECG was radiotelemetered to the base-station hospital where a physician directed therapy. Ventricular fibrillation was present when the MICU arrived. Defibrillation resulted in complete heart block, which spontaneously converted to normal sinus rhythm. The patient made a good recovery.

When cardiac arrest is present, pulmonary ventilation is maintained by use of an esophageal obturator airway (Fig. 4.8).[7,31] This device consists of a cuffed endotracheal tube mounted through a face mask and modified with a soft plastic obturator blocking the distal orifice and multiple openings in the upper one-third of the tube at the level of the pharynx. It can be passed into the esophagus with ease without direct visualization. When the cuff is inflated the regurgitation of gastric contents is prevented. If the patient remains unconscious upon arrival at the hospital, an endotracheal tube is inserted before the esophageal airway is removed.

In the case of the Los Angeles County Fire Department MICUs, it is necessary to use a private ambulance to transport the patient. One paramedic, together with the portable equipment, accompanies the patient to the hospital. Although this system has obvious disadvantages, it does permit the institution of a sophisticated MICU service at less expense, since the purchase of new vehicles is not necessary.

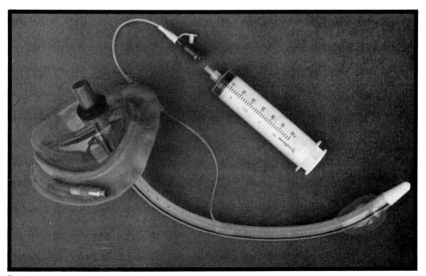

Figure 4.8
Esophageal obturator airway.

Since the hospital base-station physician is in continuous contact with the paramedic team, he is immediately prepared to take over therapy when the patient arrives at the hospital. In the case of a cardiac problem, the patient can be transported by the paramedic directly from the ambulance to the cardiac care unit with continuous monitoring.

The paramedic keeps a brief written record of each case. At the base station, all voice and ECG communications are recorded on magnetic tape. This is kept as a permanent record.

Legal aspects of MICU operation. In 1969, when the paramedic program was begun in Los Angeles County, the paramedic did not have the legal authority to defibrillate or to administer drugs. At that time it was necessary for a nurse to accompany the paramedics on each run. In July 1970, the California state legislature modified the State Health and Safety Code with the passage of the Wedworth–Townsend Paramedic Act (California Health and Safety Code, article 3, chapter 2.5, division 2).

This legislation permitted a properly trained paramedic to initiate cardiopulmonary resuscitation and to defibrillate a pulseless, nonbreathing patient. The paramedic was then required to establish radio or telephone contact with a physician (or specially certified MICU nurse) who could authorize the paramedic to start an intravenous solution and to administer parenterally any of the following six categories of drugs: antiarrhythmic agents, vagolytic agents, chronotropic agents, analgesic agents, alkalinizing agents, or vasopressor agents. In addition, the paramedic was allowed to perform gastric intubation for the prevention of aspiration.

This legislation was initially restricted to Los Angeles County to determine the feasibility of utilizing paramedics in a role traditionally reserved for physicians or nurses. In July 1971, the legislation was expanded to include the entire state.

Results achieved with mobile life-support units. It is important to view the results achieved by these units with a realistic perspective. In a summary of nine studies, Fulton and associates found that 40–75% of deaths from AMI occurred within 1 hour of symptom onset.[8] Figure 4.9 is based on a study of 64 patients with definite or probable AMI admitted to a CCU.[23] It can be seen that the greatest portion of time between the onset of symptoms and the arrival at the hospital occurs before the decision was made to call for medical assistance. The mobile LSUs can only influence AMI mortality after the call for help has been made, by instituting definitive therapy at an earlier time. A large por-

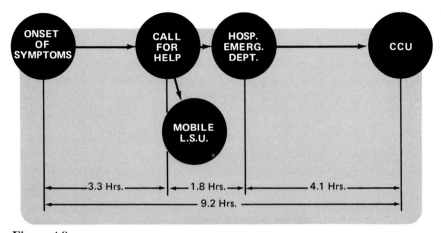

Figure 4.9
Average delay periods experienced by patients in obtaining definitive therapy for acute myocardial infarction by conventional means in 64 patients with definite or probable AMI. The potential influence of a mobile life-support unit (MLSU) is indicated. Figure is based on data from Moss.[22]

tion of AMI deaths occur, however, within 60 min of symptom onset; hence, the MCCU/MICU per se cannot be expected to reduce greatly the overall mortality.

In 1969, Pantridge and Adgey reported their experience with 61 patients with VF seen by a MCCU prior to hospitalization.[25] Thirty-nine (64%) were initially resuscitated, and 24 (39%) were long-term survivors. Resuscitation was initiated within 4 min of cardiac arrest in each of the survivors. There were no survivors among 13 more patients in whom no resuscitative measures were instituted within 4 min. Lewis and Criley in an ongoing study of the results of a mobile intensive care program encountered 246 patients with VF prior to hospitalization over a 3½-year period.[18] Seventy (28.4%) patients were resuscitated in the field and arrived at the hospital with a supraventricular rhythm. Twenty (8.1%) survived the period of hospitalization. Others have reported between 13% and 25% survivors.[6,10]

Stationary life-support units. Stationary LSUs possess the same capabilities as the mobile units but are located in areas where an acute cardiac emergency is probable or likely. This includes the hospital emergency department and certain areas out of the hospital. To evaluate effectively and manage the patient who presents with symptoms suggestive of AMI or who has sustained cardiac arrest, the following principles are essential in a hospital emergency department. These principles are based on a program of emergency room evaluation developed by the Los Angeles County Heart Association, and are in accord with the recommendations of the National Conference on Cardiopulmonary Resuscitation and Emergency Cardiac Care.[31]

1. High-priority attention must be given to patients with suspected AMI, including the institution of ECG monitoring and appropriate antiarrhythmic therapy.
2. There should be standing orders for emergency room nursing staff to initiate ECG monitoring, cardiopulmonary resuscitation, and therapy of life-threatening arrhythmias when a physician is not in immediate attendance.
3. There should be direct transfer of the patient to the CCU when he is stable. During transfer the patient should be accompanied by trained personnel using a portable ECG monitor and defibrillator.
4. There should be 24-hour daily emergency room staffing by personnel trained in the recognition and treatment of emergency cardiac problems.
5. The minimal level of training for emergency room physicians and nurses should include the recognition of life-threatening arrhythmias and their appropriate drug therapy, the performance of cardiopulmonary resuscitation, and the technique of defibrillation.
6. There should be emergency equipment and standard cardiac emergency drugs immediately available in the emergency room. This should include an ECG monitor, a defibrillator, respiratory assistance apparatus, endotracheal intubation equipment, and appropriate cardiac drugs (*i.e.*, lidocaine, atropine, isoproterenol, epinephrine, norepinephrine, sodium bicarbonate, and calcium chloride).

Stationary LSUs may also be useful outside of the hospital in areas where large numbers of people congregate, such as sport arenas,[2] convention halls, and auditoriums. They should possess the same capabilities to evaluate and treat the patient with a potential AMI or with cardiac arrest as in mobile- and hospital-based LSUs. In addition, a mobile LSU must be available to transfer the patient to the CCU.

CONCLUSIONS

To reduce the high incidence of death from coronary artery disease, attention must be focused on the patient before he reaches the sophisticated confines of the CCU. Both the physician and the patient must become aware of the prodromal symptoms of AMI and of the urgent need for instituting prompt ECG monitoring and appropriate antiarrhythmic therapy. Because of the high incidence of sudden death outside the hospital, lay persons should be instructed in basic life-support techniques (cardiopulmonary resuscitation).[31] Physicians should be required to demonstrate proficiency in basic life support. Those whose practice involves the care of cardiac patients must be proficient in the recognition and management of life-threatening arrhythmias.

REFERENCES

[1] Bondurant S: Problems of the prehospital phase of acute myocardial infarction. Am J Cardiol 24:612-616, 1969

[2] Carveth S: Cardiac resuscitation program at the Nebraska football stadium. Dis Chest 53:8–11, 1968

[3] Chiang BN, Perlman LV, Fulton M, Ostrander LD, Jr., Epstein FH: Predisposing factors in sudden cardiac death in Tecumseh, Michigan. Circulation 41:31–37, 1970

[4] Chiang BN, Perlman LV, Ostrander LD, Jr., Epstein FH: Relationship of premature systoles to coronary heart disease and sudden death in the Tecumseh epidemiologic study. Ann Intern Med 70:1159–1166, 1969

[5] Cobb LA, Conn RD, Samson WE, Philbin JE: Early experiences in the management of sudden death with a mobile intensive/coronary care unit. Circulation 42 (suppl 3): 144, 1970

[6] Cobb LA, Conn RD, Samson WE: Prehospital coronary care: The role of a rapid response mobile intensive/coronary care system. Circulation 44(supl 2): 11–45, 1971

[7] Don Michael TA, Gordon A: Esophageal airway: A new adjunct for artificial ventilation. Unpublished paper presented at the National Conference on Cardiopulmonary Resuscitation and Emergency Cardiac Care, Washington, May 16, 1973

[8] Fulton M, Julian DG, Oliver MF: Sudden death and myocardial infarction. Circulation 40(suppl 4):182–191, 1969

[9] Gazes PC, Mobley EM, Jr., Faris HM, Jr., Duncan RC, Humphries GB: Preinfarctional (unstable) angina—a prospective study—ten-year follow-up. Circulation 48:331–337, 1973

[10] Grace WJ: Coronary care: Prehospital care of acute myocardial infarction. New York, American Heart Association, 1973

[11] Grace WJ, Chadbourn JA: The mobile coronary care unit. Dis Chest 55: 452–455, 1969

[12] Kannel WB, Castelli WP, McNamara PM: The coronary profile. Twelve-year follow-up in the Framingham study. J Occup Med 9:611, 1967

[13] Kannel WB, Le Bauer EJ, Dawber TR, McNamara PM: Relation of body weight to development of coronary heart disease. Circulation 35:734–744, 1967

[14] Killip T, Kimball JT: A survey of the coronary care unit: Concept and results. Progr Cardiovasc Dis 11:45–52, 1968

[15] Kuller L: Sudden death in arteriosclerotic heart disease. Am J Cardiol 24:617–628, 1969

[16] Lawrie DM: Ventricular fibrillation in acute myocardial infarction. Am Heart J 78:424–426, 1969

[17] Lewis AJ, Ailshie G, Criley JM: Prehospital cardiac care in a paramedical mobile intensive care unit. Calif Med 117:1–8, 1972

[18] Lewis AJ, Criley JM: Unpublished data

[19] Lewis RP, Frazier JT, Warren JV: An approach to the early mortality of myocardial infarction. AM J Cardiol 26:644, 1970

[20] Lown B, Klein MD, Hershberg PI: Coronary and precoronary care. Am J Med 46:705–724, 1969

[21] Lown B, Ruberman W: The concept of precoronary care. Mod Concepts Cardiovasc Dis 39:97–102, 1970

[22] Moss AJ, Goldstein S: The prehospital phase of acute myocardial infarction. Circulation 41:737–742, 1970

[23] Moss AJ, Wynar B, Goldstein S: Delay in hospitalization during the acute coronary period. Am J Cardiol 24:659–665, 1969

[24] Nagel EL, Hirschman JC, Nussenfeld SR, Rankin D, Lundblad E: Telemetry—medical command in coronary and other mobile emergency care systems. JAMA 214:332–338, 1970

[25] Pantridge JF, Adgey AAJ: Prehospital coronary care. Am J Cardiol 24: 666–673, 1969

[26] Pantridge JF, Geddes JS: A mobile intensive care unit in the management of myocardial infarction. Lancet 2:271–273, 1967

[27] Paul O, Schatz M: On sudden death. Circulation 43:7–10, 1971

[28] Prinzmetal M, Ekmekci A, Kennamer R, Kivoczynski JK, Shubin H, Toyoshima H: Variant form of angina pectoris. JAMA 174: 1794–1800, 1960

[29] Rose LB, Press E: Cardiac defibrillation by ambulance attendants. JAMA 219:63–68, 1972

[30] Solomon HA, Edwards AL, Killip T: Prodromata in acute myocardial infarction. Circulation 40:463–471, 1969

[31] Standards for cardiopulmonary resuscitation (CPR) and emergency cardiac care (ECC). JAMA (suppl) 227:833–868, 1974

[32] Vital Statistics of the United States. Vol. II, Part B, Table 7–116, Washington, Department of Health, Education, and Welfare, 1966

[33] Yu PN: Prehospital care of acute myocardial infarction. Circulation 45: 189–204, 1972

Neil L. Chayet

5

Medicolegal Implications
of Emergency Care

As this chapter is written, members of the medical profession and the hospitals in which they practice are in serious difficulty. Malpractice rates have never been higher for hospitals and physicians alike and reports are circulating that coverage in certain high-risk specialties will be completely unavailable this spring. Thus, it is more important than ever before that the physician and hospital personnel be aware of the proper handling of the sudden emergency so that quality care can be given and unnecessary legal risks can be avoided.

This chapter will view the responsibilities of the medical profession and the hospital in handling the emergency victim from the moment he or she is stricken until the moment of death or discharge from the hospital. Regardless of the position the reader occupies, be it physician, nurse, physician's assistant, or hospital administrator, all bear a common responsibility to see to it that the victim of an accident or sudden illness receives the best possible care at the scene, the most appropriate conveyance to a hospital, and quality care at the institution—all in a manner that maximizes proper patient care and that minimizes legal risks along the way.

AT THE SCENE

The author offered $25 for documentation of a single case in which a physician has been sued for providing emergency medical care at the scene of an accident or sudden illness. Rumors continue to abound; however, no cases have yet been documented.

The same is true to my knowledge for all other medical professionals, including nurses and physician's assistants. Nor am I aware of any cases that have been brought against police officers, fire fighters, physician's assistants, ambulance attendants, or laymen in general. In addition to there being no reported cases, I am not aware of any such cases that may have been settled out of court by insurance companies or by the individuals themselves.

In short, it is safe to say that regardless of the legal hazards that physicians face in their offices, in hospital emergency wards, and throughout the hospital in general (and they are considerable, as will be seen shortly), the concern over legal liability for actions *at the scene* is wholly unjustified.

One might question why the great fear continues. One reason is that the media continues, although with somewhat less frequency, to exploit the theme of the young physician who stops at an accident, saves a life, and as thanks ends up in a law suit. With litigation at an all-time high, and with Good Samaritans in rather short supply, the theme is a natural for television and magazines and, unfortunately, large numbers of physicians and others called upon to render such aid are besieged and affected by this material.

There are, unfortunately, other reasons why people choose not to stop at accidents. At a meeting at which the new cardiopulmonary resuscitation standards were being discussed in Atlanta a few years ago, I heard a violent crash, went to the window, and saw that a bus had hit a car that had overturned, spilling two of its occupants into the street. One was lying face down in the roadway. A policeman was already at the scene, directing traffic and talking on his walkie-talkie, but paying absolutely no attention to the injured person. I informed the doctors of what had occurred, and we rushed to the street where one of the doctors began to work with the injured. He was ordered away from the victim by the police officer who said a special squad was on the way—and it was trained in ESP!

An even more disturbing reason for not giving such aid surfaced after a recent speech on the subject of emergency care. One of the doctors in the audience approached and asked if he could see me for a moment out of the hearing of the others. When we had moved a considerable distance away from the group he stated, "Do you know why I don't stop? I don't know what to do!" Following that rather surprising admission, the curricula of several leading medical schools was reviewed and it was found that in most medical schools the teaching of the proper handling of trauma is woefully inadequate.

It is clear that better training in the area of proper rendering of emergency medical care by physicians and, in fact, by all persons is extremely necessary. One looks to the day when in-depth training in the handling of accidents and emergencies will be the rule rather than the exception; if some high schools around the country require their students to learn to swim before graduation, there is no reason why proper medical handling of emergencies could not also become a mandatory part of the curriculum.

At present, all states offer some sort of Good-Samaritan protection by statute. Most of the statutes require that the individual to receive the protection act gratuitously and in a manner that is not reckless or wanton or otherwise indicative of bad faith. These laws are not really necessary, however, because a case has never been reported against a Good Samaritan.

It was thought that the passage of such legislation, in addition to providing protection if there ever should be a suit, would also be useful in an educational sense to encourage people—physicians and others—to render aid when they came across an accident or sudden illness. In fact this has not been as effective as hoped, and a great deal of reluctance is still present, particularly among physicians and nurses who presumably are best able to cope with such situations.

Only one state, Vermont, has attempted to deal with this problem in an interesting manner; Vermont has the only Good-Samaritan law with a twist—a mandatory duty to render aid. The statute states that failure to render aid to a person in need will be fined as a criminal violation, if such aid could have been rendered without danger and without interference with important duties to others (to protect the surgeon who is en route to another case, for example). Such statutes are common in Europe but hitherto have been nonexistent in the United States where our "every-man-for-himself" philosophy has not fostered the development of a mandatory duty to help others.

Another pattern has also emerged in recent years. Statutes are being established that require persons who are regularly involved in the initial handling of emergencies to be better trained. An example is the California legislation requiring all police officers to be trained in giving cardiopulmonary resuscitation. The genesis of this legislation is interesting. It is reported that one of the California legislators had a heart attack and died; it was rumored that he might have lived if any of the police officers who initially responded had known how to perform cardiopulmonary resuscitation. Apparently the every-man-for-himself principle occasionally has some beneficial spinoff as well!

As yet, the legal difficulties of on-the-scene handling of medical emergencies are unresolved. The most significant of these are called to mind by the incident of the American cardiologist from Cape Cod, Massachusetts, who was vacationing in the Virgin Islands. The doctor noticed a commotion on the dock, left his hotel room to see if he could help, and, when he arrived at the dock, found that a man had been electrocuted while using a power drill. The doctor tried to revive him but could not, and, as a last-ditch measure, he opened the man's chest and massaged his heart to no avail.

Rumor had it that this doctor was sued for $200,000 by the family of the victim; in fact, the doctor was never sued. Rather, he was thanked for his efforts by the family. Unfortunately, the story does not end there. Although he was not sued, he was arrested for practicing medicine without a license, preliminary to a charge of murder that was to be lodged against him following the results of an autopsy. After the intervention of the President of the United States (John Kennedy), the physician was allowed to return home, much shaken from his sole experience as a Good Samaritan. This problem is the unlawful practice of medicine or violation of the medical practice acts of a given jurisdiction.

A Good-Samaritan act may pose a problem for a physician who is traveling through a jurisdiction in which he is not licensed or for the police officer, fire fighter, ambulance attendant, or layman who is called upon to take immediate action. Most jurisdictions in the United States have exceptions in their medical-practice acts for emergency situations, but there is some question whether or not a paramedic who rides an ambulance 4 nights a week in areas where emergencies are regularly anticipated would qualify for such an exemption.

Some experts in the field believe that the medical-practice acts require that telemetry actually connect the physician with the person who is going to operate a defibrillator or start intravenous (I-V) treatment. Development of model legislation is clearly needed that will assure appropriate training in areas of greatest need and that will afford a measure of protection for those involved in the rendering of emergency medical care at the scene.

CONVEYANCE OF THE ILL OR INJURED

It is hoped that some day in the not-too-distant future a person who is stricken with a heart attack, for example, will receive immediate and proper care from a layman who has had training in cardiopulmonary resuscitation, then care from a well-trained responder—a police officer or fire fighter—and when indicated, defibrillation and I-V therapy from a well-trained emergency medical technician who is operating a well-equipped secondary response vehicle. When stabilized, the patient will be conveyed to an appropriate receiving facility with which the vehicle has been in constant communication, and the victim will then receive continuous and intensive care at this facility or at another more specialized facility to which he or she may be transferred. Unfortunately, we are a very long distance from this idyllic set of circumstances in nearly all sections of the country.

The more typical response is similar to that recounted to me by a Massachusetts psychiatrist who was willing to be a Good Samaritan but was unprepared for the events that followed. While driving on a rural highway, he came across a car stopped by the side of the road. A man was slumped over the hood of the car and a woman was standing by him, patiently waiting for some assistance. The psychiatrist stopped and asked the woman if she needed help. She said the man, whom she identified as her husband, was simply having another asthma attack "like the one he had last spring."

It turned out that the family doctor had not wanted to worry her, so when her husband had had a nearly fatal heart attack last spring, he told her it was merely an asthma attack. The doctor, however, recognized that her husband was indeed having a heart attack; he managed to get him in the back of his car and after about 10 min of searching, found a pay telephone. He dialed the operator and was transferred to the police who responded, "We don't handle that stuff. Call the fire department," and hung up. The doctor then dialed information, got the number for the fire department, and finally reached a man who said he wished he could be of help, "but our vehicle is busy right now at a fire," and he gave the doctor directions to the nearest hospital. "It's easy to get to," he said, "Just follow the blue signs," which led the doctor, after about 30 min on a picturesque New England road, to a hospital that no longer had an emergency room. In desperation, the doctor called the state police, who responded 20 min later with a station wagon, by which time the man had died, a victim of an almost total failure of what is euphemistically called the "Emergency Medical Care System."

The first major piece of federal legislation that was passed in the area of emergency medical services, PL 93–154, holds some hope of bringing badly needed federal funding and direction to an area that for the most part is chaotic and inefficient, causing each year needless death and more serious injury to thousands of ill and injured. One need only stand by the doorway of almost any major emergency department and watch the manner in which the ill and injured are shuttled to and fro.

The act provides for pilot funding (although there are internal governmental squabbles about the manner and under whose direction the monies will be disbursed) to regional or other programs which meet the following criteria:[1]

(i)   include an adequate number of health professions, allied health professions, and other health personnel with appropriate training and experience;

(ii)   provide for its personnel appropriate training (including clinical training) and continuing education programs which (I) are coordinated with other programs in the system's service area which provide similar training and education, and (II) emphasize recruitment and necessary training of veterans of the Armed Forces with military training and experience in health care fields and of appropriate public safety personnel in such area;

(iii)   join the personnel, facilities, and equipment of the system by a central communications system so that requests for emergency health care services will be handled by a communications facility which (I) utilizes emergency medical telephonic screening, (II) utilizes or, within such period as the Secretary prescribes will utilize, the universal emergency telephone number 911, and (III) will have direct communication connections and interconnections with the personnel, facilities, and equipment of the system and with other appropriate emergency medical services systems;

(iv)   include an adequate number of necessary ground, air, and water vehicles and other transportation facilities to meet the individual characteristics of the system's service area,

(a)   which vehicles and facilities meet appropriate standards relating to location, design, performance, and equipment, and

(b)   the operators and other personnel for which vehicles and facilities meet appropriate training and experience requirements;

(v)   include an adequate number of easily accessible emergency medical services facilities which are collectively capable of providing services on a continuous basis, which have appropriate nonduplicative and categorized capabilities, which meet appropriate standards relating to capacity, location, personnel, and equipment, and which are coordinated with other health care facilities of the system;

(vi) provide access (including appropriate transportation) to specialized critical medical care units in the system's service area, or, if there are no such units or an inadequate number of them in such area, provide access to such units in neighboring areas if access to such units is feasible in terms of time and distance;

(vii) provide for the effective utilization of the appropriate personnel, facilities, and equipment of each public safety agency providing emergency services in the system's service area;

(viii) be organized in such a manner that provides persons who reside in the system's service area and who have no professional training or financial interest in the provision of health care with an adequate opportunity to participate in the making of policy for the system;

(ix) provide, without prior inquiry as to ability to pay, necessary emergency medical services to all patients requiring such services;

(x) provide for transfer of patients to facilities and programs which offer such follow-up care and rehabilitation as is necessary to effect the maximum recovery of the patient;

(xi) provide for a standardized patient recordkeeping system meeting appropriate standards established by the Secretary, which records shall cover the treatment of the patient from initial entry into the system through his discharge from it, and shall be consistent with ensuing patient records used in follow-up care and rehabilitation of the patient;

(xii) provide programs of public education and information in the system's service area (taking into account the needs of visitors to, as well as residents of that area to know or be able to learn immediately how to obtain emergency medical services) which programs stress the general dissemination of information regarding appropriate methods of medical self-help and first-aid and regarding the availability of first-aid training programs in the area;

(xiii) provide for (I) periodic, comprehensive, and independent review and evaluation of the extent and quality of the emergency health care services provided in the system's service area, and (II) submission to the Secretary of the reports of each such review and evaluation;

(xiv) have a plan to assure that the system will be capable of providing emergency medical services in the system's service area during mass casualties, natural disasters, or national emergencies; and

(xv) provide for the establishment of appropriate arrangements with emergency medical services systems or similar entities serving neighboring areas for the provision of emergency medical services on a reciprocal basis where access to such services would be more appropriate and effective in terms of the services available, time, and distance.

ARRIVAL AT THE HOSPITAL; END OF SOME WOES; BEGINNING OF OTHERS

A well-defined plan for emergency care, based on community need and on the capability of the hospital, shall exist within every hospital . . . The hospital must have some procedure whereby the ill or injured person can be assessed, and either treated or referred to an appropriate facility, as indicated. Most hospitals that offer a broad range of services can provide effective care for any type of patient requiring emergency service. Hospitals that offer a partial range of services may be capable of operating a limited emergency service only, and, therefore, must arrange for the transfer or referral of certain patients to other institutions. Some hospitals may elect to refer all emergency patients. In either case, the referring hospital must institute essential lifesaving measures and provide emergency procedures that will minimize aggravation of the condition during transportation. Inherent in this action is the understanding that no patient should arbitrarily be transferred if the hospital where he was initially seen has means for adequate care of his problem. The patient may not be transferred until the receiving institution has consented to accept that patient. A reasonable record of the immediate medical problem must accompany the patient.

The hospital and its medical staff should promote, and help develop, a community-based emergency plan, and should show evidence of such participation. The degree to which a hospital provides emergency care should be guided by the community plan.

The quotation is from the "Standards of the Joint Commission on Accreditation."[2] One might question the advisability of every hospital having capability for dealing with emergencies in some manner. Since the problem often stems from the public being misled about the presence or absence of emergency capability, one might have suggested that a hospital need not have emergency capability if it publicized this fact adequately.

Under the quoted standard, every hospital must have a means of dealing with emergencies. The interpretation of the standard indicates a responsibility for transfer of those cases that cannot be competently handled at the hospital, and all hospitals should have a clearly defined plan for expeditiously dealing with such cases.

Similarly all hospitals should keep in mind the case of *Brune* v. *Belinkoff*, which for all intents and purposes abolished the locality standard of care.[3] Formerly, hospitals, as well as physicians, were responsible for providing care that was no better and no worse than that available in the geographic area in which they were located. This case, which has now been cited as authority across the nation, stated that

> Distinctions based on geography are no longer valid in view of modern developments, transportation, communication, and medical education, all of which tend to promote a certain degree of standardization in the profession. Today with the rapid methods of transportation and easy means of communication, the horizons have been widened and the duty of a doctor is not fulfilled merely by utilizing the means at hand in the particular village where he is practicing. So far as medical treatment is concerned, the borders of the locality and community have in effect been extended so as to include those centers readily accessible where appropriate treatment may be had which the local physician, because of limited facilities or training, is unable to give.. . . The time has come when the medical profession should no longer be Balkanized by the allegation of varying geographic standards in malpractice cases.[3]

Although it is now clear that all hospitals must have the capability for dealing with emergencies, many nagging questions remain. One of the most difficult is deciding when an emergency is in fact present. It is a well-known fact that with the changing relationships between physicians and their patients and the decreasing availability of physicians on evenings and weekends, many people seek help at emergency rooms for situations that, in the minds of many emergency room physicians and nurses, do not qualify as *bona fide* emergencies.

Very little guidance is available from the courts in answering this question. The classic case is the *Wilmington General Hospital* v. *Manlove*.[4] This case is usually cited for the principle that persons needing emergency care cannot be turned away from a facility that publicizes the fact that emergency care is available at the facility. The court cited as its reasoning that, if a person needing emergency care arrived at a facility that had an "Emergency Room" sign and was then turned away, the patient has lost valuable time and possibly would suffer damage as a result. This well-known aspect of the case is reinforced by the standards and interpretations of the joint commission as previously cited.

The questions of the manner in which the emergency room is staffed and the manner in which responsibility for patient care is discharged are of supreme importance from both a legal and medical point of view. There are basically four methods of staffing emergency rooms. One is by forcing a rotation of all staff members through the emergency room.

This method is not employed very much today, and it is just as well, for it has often resulted in physicians manning the emergency room with virtually no expertise in handling trauma or sudden illness. If this method is employed, hospital administration must be certain that any physician who is responsible for the emergency room is trained to deal with emergencies that may occur during his time of duty.

A second method of staffing is to utilize residents from teaching hospitals to supplement the staff handling the emergency room. Even though this method is preferable to the first method, it leaves a good deal to be desired, and if utilized, caution must be taken to have available prompt consultative assistance by other competent staff members.

The third and fourth methods involve full-time emergency-room physicians. The third is by physicians who are employees of the hospital or a corporation that contracts with the hospital and that in turn employs the emergency-room physicians. This is by far the best method of staffing an emergency room. It is not, however, without its problems. In this method it is essential that a carefully drawn contract is made between the emergency-room physicians or the corporation of which they are a part and the hospital to clarify their financial and professional relationship. Such a contract should also incorporate by reference hospital regulations that clarify the relationship between the emergency-room physician and the staff physician.

The problem is twofold. What is the relationship between the emergency-room physician when the patient of another physician seeks assistance and what is the responsibility of the consultant staff physician in a given specialty when he is summoned by the emergency-room physician?

Hospital regulations should make it clear that the emergency-room physician is responsible for every patient who enters the emergency room. The staff physician who may have treated the patient previously should be notified and, of course, may come to the emergency room and assume treatment of the patient if he wishes. The main point, however, is that the emergency-room physician retains medical and legal responsibility for the patient until the attending physician physically arrives at the hospital.

Furthermore, the emergency-room physician should have admitting privileges. When he deems it appropriate after the initial evaluation, the emergency-room physician should be able to admit the patient to the hospital. The attending physician who has treated the patient in the past or a physician selected on a rotation basis should be notified of the admission. The emergency-room physician, however, maintains responsibility for the patient until the attending physician actually arrives and notes his arrival on the patient's chart. This procedure avoids the possibility of conflicting telephone orders and the virtual abandonment of the patient by physicians between the time of admission and arrival of the attending doctor.

CONCLUSION

In summary, great strides have been made over the last several years in the care of the victim at the scene, conveyance to a facility, and care at the receiving hospital. Nevertheless, a great deal remains to be done, and it will take the cooperation of medical, legal, and political forces to bring about the level of emergency medical care that we expect and deserve.

REFERENCES

[1] Emergency Medical Services Act of 1973. Public Law 93–154, Washington, 93rd Congress of the U. S., 1973

[2] Standards of the Joint Commission on Accreditation. Accreditation Manual for Hospitals. Hospital Accreditation Program, Chicago, JCAH, 1971, p.71

[3] Brune v. Belinkoff, 354 Mass 102; 235 NE 2d 793 (1968)

[4] Wilmington General Hospital v. Manlove, 174 A2d 135

II

Prehospital

John M. Waters

6

Field Treatment and Transportation

GENERAL CRITERIA

In establishing criteria for field treatment and transport, we must define the role they will play. If the ambulance is merely used as a convalescent or chronic-patient transport vehicle carrying patients not requiring immediate treatment, the equipment and training needed would be only minimal. At the other end of the spectrum are the highly specialized vehicles and crews generally reserved for special cases such as heart attacks and that receive relatively limited use for the high monetary investment involved.

Realistically, most ambulances must be used for both purposes, especially when operated by commercial or volunteer organizations, and should therefore carry adequate equipment and trained manpower to deal with life-threatening emergencies, even though such cases are only a fraction of the total. Some of the more advanced municipally operated systems triage and diagnose in the field and only transport cases deemed to be of an urgent or emergency nature; such a procedure more quickly frees the involved unit to return to service, and nonemergency patients can be transported to a medical facility by private conveyance or nonemergency private ambulance.

DETECTION AND DECISION DELAY

The greatest delay in getting definitive care for the patient most often involves a delay in the call for help, for the most responsive emergency system cannot act until it is alerted. In terms of numbers and mortality, the less serious of these delays involve discovery of an accident victim, usually in the home or on the highway. These accidents may involve older persons living or working alone or highway travelers on roads that are used infrequently during the late night hours. Despite discussions about sophisticated crash locator beacons and alerting devices, economics make their use in automobiles prohibitive, and the passerby must be relied on to spread the alarm. Excessive delays are not common.

A far more serious problem involves delay in calling for help following onset of cardiac symptoms. Delays of 3–6 hours after onset are common. As the period of greatest danger is the first 1–3 hours after onset and the heart attack is the greatest killer in this country, it is not surprising that over half of all heart attack deaths occur before reaching a physician. In view of the extremely critical time element, with irreversible damage occurring within 3–5 min after cardiac arrest, the necessity of the earliest possible call for help should be starkly apparent. Should cardiac arrest occur before help arrives, the only hope for the victim is the immediate presence of one or more persons capable of giving cardiopulmonary resuscitation.

The elimination of decision delay for heart attack victims is not merely one of education, but probably involves a psychological denial syndrome, *i.e.,* "This can't be happening to me!"

This tendency suggests that education must strongly emphasize not only the symptoms but also that a prompt call can activate a system to save the victim. It must also stress that the emergency response system is there for that purpose and rescue personnel do not consider a call as an imposition.

WHO TO CALL

Ironically, there appear to be more facilities potentially capable of rendering some type of emergency medical care than the dispatching centers and answering services are able to contact and control. This fact is largely due to fractionalization and parochialism in establishing the communication center or Emergency Operating Center (EOC). Such EOCs may vary in complexity from a major city police or fire center to the office of a rural county sheriff located at the jail with one person running the operation. The person seeking help is usually in a quandary, unless he has local knowledge, because of the multiplicity of townships, counties, and other political entities, with dozens of different jurisdictions within a small area and each with its own control center or centers. The consumer may be forced to run his finger through the Yellow Pages and play a dangerous game of roulette with his own life as the stake.

We must submerge parochial interests to the common good by establishing regional centers that can service a large area containing many different political jurisdictions and facilities. Such centers may be for medical emergencies only, but they would be more effective as public safety EOCs, controlling not only medical units, but also police and fire units. Whether the ambulance providers are public, commercial, or volunteer is immaterial; such a public safety center can dispatch medical help efficiently, including backup police, fire, and wrecker service. Such centers do not diminish the authority of the individual police or fire chief or ambulance operator, but they act as a service bureau to them, while effecting substantial monetary savings. The proven success of a number of such regional centers only emphasize the waste and obsoleteness of dozens of separate competing and inadequate small answering locations within the same area.

HOW TO CALL

Nearly all calls for help will be by commercial telephone. How to reach a source of help is a major problem, and the establishment of regional centers or joint public safety centers is a *sine qua non* for assignment of a common phone number. The most popular trend now is toward the use of the common emergency number, 911. While its adoption would be a highly desirable national goal, numerous technical and fiscal problems remain. The lack of common telephone company and political boundaries is one of the major ones, but this can be eased by the regional concept. Many fire chiefs and ambulance operators fear that the quality with which they service calls will be lessened by the very high volume of police calls coming in on 911. Most of these police calls will be trivial complaints and not of an emergency nature. It is interesting to note that in a typical metropolitan area, nearly one-third of all *real* emergency calls involve medical problems, although 90% of all calls on the switchboard are directed to the police.

81

Next to 911, perhaps the most effective method is the placing of gummed emergency number stickers on all phones. Printing of emergency numbers in the inside front cover of the phone book is effective to some extent, but is largely nullified if there are dozens of emergency numbers in one metropolitan area phone book due to lack of a regional center. Dialing the operator for help is often effective; if she is indecisive, ask her to connect you with the nearest fire or police department. Far down the list of alternatives is selecting an ambulance from the Yellow Pages.

We should view with some skepticism the advice often given, even by such authoritative organizations as the American Heart Association, such as, "Call your doctor. If you are unable to reach him, go to a hospital immediately." The fallacies inherent here are obvious. What is the average delay in reaching your doctor, assuming you have a personal physician? Failing this, does this advice imply that you load the coronary patient or trauma victim with shattered limb in a vehicle and speed to the nearest hospital? In a community with even a fair emergency medical system, the obvious answer is that the response by the ambulance and public safety agency will be far faster than that of a physician. The patient can be delivered to an emergency department, where the physician is in a proper setting to treat the critical patient. It also seems obvious that a critically ill patient in a properly equipped rescue ambulance is in better position to survive a setback than he would be in the back seat of a private vehicle. The specter of a coronary patient driving himself to a hospital at 90 miles per hour needs no comment. If a community must rely on calling a physician and getting the critical patient to a hospital without rescue ambulance and public safety help, it is indeed a dangerous place to live.

The difficulty of obtaining access to the emergency medical system due to the lack of planning and regionalization presents one of the biggest obstacles to emergency health delivery care today. Regional planning would not only significantly reduce this problem but would also effectively reduce the cost of maintaining communication and control facilities.

ADAPTIVE RESPONSE

The response by the center receiving the call for help will depend on its evaluation of the situation. This situation may involve a prank call or one of no urgent need, or the call may be the first indication of a disaster situation. In any case, as long as an emergency exists in the mind of the caller, it must be treated as such until trained personnel can arrive on the scene and properly evaluate it. A serious accident or a myocardial infarction call for an all-out initial response that could involve a rescue ambulance, a fire company, and a police car. Such a multiple dispatch affords fast access as well as manpower, and both are needed in serious cases. Fire and police personnel, most of whom have at least basic first-aid training, constitute perhaps the greatest untapped source of emergency medical care (EMC), and their participation is a keystone of such outstanding emergency systems as those in Jacksonville, Florida; Seattle, Washington; Houston, Texas; and Miami, Florida.

VEHICULAR EQUIPMENT

An emergency (rescue) ambulance must be able to proceed safely through congested traffic at above average traffic speeds, while braking and accelerating as required to pass intersections and other vehicles safely. Handling characteristics should also provide for good cornering and quick evasion turns. Although high-speed runs with lights and siren are rarely required from the scene of the accident to the hospital if the patient is properly stabilized, they do occur with regularity en route to the scene, when time is often a critical factor.

The vehicle should have a body with adequate space to contain all required equipment as well as room to work on the patient. The equipment carried should conform to the allowed medical practices by paramedical personnel in each state; there is no rationale for carrying equipment that personnel are neither allowed nor trained to use. The size and type of vehicle will thus depend on the equipment carried and the procedures allowed under existing medical practice.

The lists of essential equipment for ambulances outlined by the National Research Council, National Academy of Sciences[5] and that published by the American College of Surgeons[2] is generally considered quite adequate for the existing standards of care in most areas of the country today. The latter document recognizes that changes in care are occurring rapidly and anticipates that future requirements will generally include drug-injection kits, defibrillators with cardioscopes, radio and telephone ECG telemetry capability, venous cut-down kit, etc. Extrication equipment is recommended for those rescue ambulances not accompanied by a fire company or other specially trained extrication team. Whenever possible, heavy extrication should be left to a fire department ladder company or heavy rescue company, while the emergency medical technicians (EMTs) concentrate on immobilization and care of the patient during extrication.

AMBULANCE TYPES

The past 7 years have seen a great surge of interest in ambulance design and equipment due in large measure to the impetus of the National Highway Safety Act of 1966 and the emphasis on EMC generated by that act. In 1970, the National Research Council, National Academy of Sciences published "Medical Requirements for Ambulance Design and Equipment," which set the broad medical criteria for further ambulance development and equipment categories. These general requirements were translated into specific engineering design standards by the National Academy of Engineering with the publication of "Ambulance Design Criteria" in May 1971.[1] Compliance with these standards was made mandatory in volume 11 of the Highway Safety Programs Manual for any person expending federal funds for ambulance procurement. The General Services Administration has also put out minimum specifications for procurement of ambulances for the federal government.

There are four major types of ambulances in use today in the United States. They are the automobile type, the carryall (large station wagon), the van type, and the modular type.

The automobile type (Fig. 6.1) consists of an ambulance body constructed upon a standard or lengthened automobile chassis. Although historically common and still very prevalent in the country, such a vehicle cannot meet the space standards required by the new criteria and is usually unable to carry all required equipment. The regular (small) station wagon converted for ambulance use is even more restricted and is totally unsuitable for emergency use. It seems apparent that the automobile-type ambulance, due to its restrictions and high

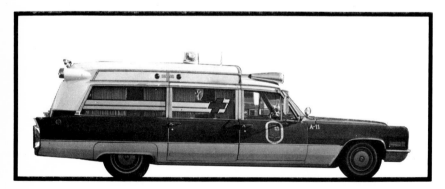

Figure 6.1
The hearse-type ambulance. This vehicle cannot meet space requirements and is unable to carry all necessary equipment.

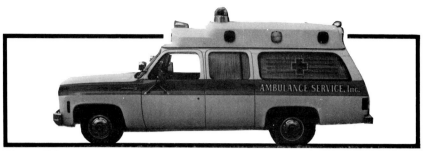

Figure 6.2
The carryall ambulance on a truck-type chassis. These vehicles have difficulty meeting space criteria, and their use is diminishing.

initial costs, will rapidly disappear from the scene as the present models reach replacement age and are unlikely to figure prominently in the future in emergency vehicle plans.

Figure 6.2 shows the carryall ambulance, constructed on a standard truck-type chassis. The van type ambulance (Fig. 6.3), because of its body style, offers considerably more inside room than either of the preceding two types. Although it has a roomy patient compartment, its overall length and wheelbase are the shortest of any of the four types being compared.

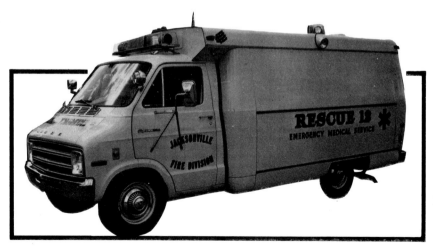

Figure 6.3
The van-type ambulance with ample cabin space. The chassis is not changeable.

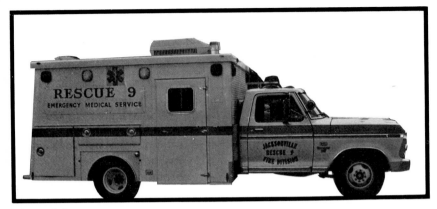

Figure 6.4
Modular ambulance with all-aluminum body. Note numerous exterior compartments and the commercial-type air conditioner on top of cabin.

The modular unit (Fig. 6.4), has been rapidly gaining acceptance throughout the country, especially by the larger city-operated departments providing advanced sophisticated care and running thousands of cases, the result being heavy chassis wear. The patient compartment is essentially a box mounted on a 1-ton truck cab and chassis. When the chassis is worn out after lengthy service, the box is lifted off and placed on a new chassis at a cost considerably below the usual vehicle replacement cost. The patient compartment meets all space requirements and can carry all required equipment to treat the critically injured or ill patient in the field. Figure 6.5 shows the interior of one of these modular units operated by the Jacksonville Fire Division.

Comparisons of the four types of ambulances were made by Garrett in March 1973.[3] These costs, corrected to 1975 standards, are based on replacing three types of the vehicles every 3 years and replacing the chassis of the fourth or modular type every 3 years, with one body lasting through three chassis changes. Table 6.1 clearly indicates cost and space advantages of the modular (truck) unit. In areas of light usage, however, ambulances last longer, and the chassis-change feature of the modular unit is less advantageous.

Additional equipment requirements (Table 6.2) were computed by Garrett[3] and updated by Waters.

The primary disadvantage cited for the modular type is its rough ride. Although this is certainly true, it is essential to note that with proper stabilization of patients on the scene, only 10% of runs from the scene of the accident to the hospital are made at high speeds by units of the

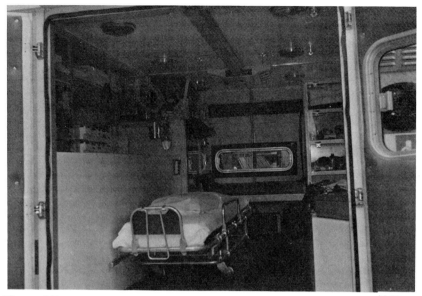

Figure 6.5
Interior of a modular unit containing both interior and exterior compartments. This unit carries equipment for nearly any emergency.

Jacksonville Fire Division, and at these slower speeds and with proper patient stabilization and immobilization, the rough ride is of far less significance; in terms of space, only the van type is comparable to the modular unit. The van has received much criticism, however, about its safety because of the forward location of the driver and some criticism about its stability. For communities having few annual runs and delivering basic emergency medical care, the van is as suitable as the modular unit and just as cost-effective.

The large special purpose units, such as the mobile coronary care units, have not been discussed, as they serve no real need that would justify their added expense, cumbersome handling, and limited use. The modular unit is fully capable of providing both the space and the equipment to handle a coronary or other acute case. It is operationally impractical to provide one or two units to handle a special type of case when one considers that such cases constitute perhaps 10% of all calls, and they can be handled in any event by smaller and more cost-effective units. Rather than the mobile coronary care unit, which is concerned only with the coronary patient, we should think of the mobile life-support unit, which deals with all emergency patients.

Table 6.1. Vehicle Comparison

Type	Typical cost (new)*	Depreciation per year (9-year basis)	Advantages	Disadvantages
Automobile Cadillac chassis	$22,000	$5,100	Good ride	Small patient area (does not meet space criteria; small storage capacity; poor off-highway vehicle; low maneuverability
Carryall Springfield equipment model 149 (Int'l Harv. chassis)	12,600	2,740	Good off-road vehicle (4-wheel drive option readily available)	Cannot meet patient area criteria; relatively harsh ride
Van Superior (Chevy G-30 chassis) or Wayne Carovan	13,500	3,113	Large patient area; large storage capacity; good maneuverability	No 4-wheel drive option for off-highway use; relatively harsh ride
Modular Swab Eagle 120 (Ford F-350 chassis) or modulance	14,500	2,220	Large patient area; large storage capacity; good off-road vehicle (with special chassis)	Harsh ride

*Approximate list prices as of 1975.

Table 6.2. Equipment Requirements

Equipment	Cost*	Total cost
Mobile 4-channel UHF transceiver	$1,500	
Defibrillator-electrocardioscope	4,000	
Portable UHF voice/telemetry transceiver	3,000	
		$8,500
Portable oxygen equipment with masks	200	
Oxygen bottles—portable (2) and vehicle-mounted (1)	100	
Portable suction (foot-powered) (option: battery-powered portable suction @ $1,851)	50	
		350
Airways and bag masks	170	
Bandages, dressings, etc.	60	
Blankets, pillows, sheets, sterile sheets, etc.	75	
Blood pressure manometer and stethoscope	40	
Esophageal airways	60	
I-V administration kits, agents, and drugs	120	
Medical bag and drug kit	70	
Miscellaneous instruments, services, and supplies	70	
Obstetric kit	10	
Poison kit	10	
Spine boards (long and short) and accessories	100	
Splints (half-ring; moulded wood GI; padded board)	150	
Trousers antishock (MAST)	300†	
		1,235
120 vs 3,000 W inverter with outlets	700	
Fire extinguisher	50	
Power jack (4-ton)	250	
Rope: 50 ft × ¾ in. (2)	25	
Extrication hand tools	130	1,155
		$11,240

* Approximate list prices as of 1975.
† Estimated cost.

OTHER ASSISTING UNITS

Ambulances should be strategically located after a careful analysis of workload, time–distance factors, and basic queuing probability study. These dispositions may very well change at different times of the day as the populations shifts between residential and business districts. Even with optimal placement of units, however, assistance from other agencies may be needed to provide an earlier arriving source of help or additional manpower to handle a case. The primary resource agencies are the fire and police departments. Because they are able to move rapidly through traffic in territory which is familiar to them, these public safety units will often arrive at the scene before an ambulance and can render lifesaving aid until the more sophisticated rescue ambulance arrives. In Jacksonville, Florida, where this concept has long been in force, rescue ambulances are accompanied by fire units in 40% of cases and by police in 24%.

Of perhaps equal importance is the manpower provided by police and fire fighters in handling an automobile accident or heart attack victim. In nearly all such cases, several men are needed. Public safety personnel should be (and usually are) trained in first aid and cardiopulmonary resuscitation, and most carry first-aid kits. No emergency medical service system can really be cost-effective unless fire and police personnel are an integral part of the team, regardless of who provides ambulance service.

FIELD TREATMENT

On arrival at the scene, the EMT must first make a thorough and rapid assessment of the situation, triaging the patients, and communicating with the hospital when necessary about treatment of the patients in more critical conditions. Most runs involve only one patient. After an initial check for life-threatening conditions, a brief history and vital signs are obtained. A preliminary impression is reached and confirmed if necessary with the hospital. A case history, ECGs, and other vital signs are an aid in such diagnosis. Treatment may be initiated at the discretion of the EMT or as prescribed by a physician by radio or telephone. Emphasis must be on stabilization before transportation. In advanced systems in which this is done, only 10% of runs from the scene to the hospital are done at high speed with lights and siren.

The question of which patients to transport is an operational, a medical, a political, and in the case of private service, an economic decision. With well-trained and equipped EMTs, a large percentage of patients can be initially treated in the field; then delivered to a physician or hospital by means other than ambulance. Long experience in the advanced Jacksonville system has shown that only 40% of all calls require transport by rescue ambulance; another 21% are taken to the hospital by either police or private car after field treatment.

Such a procedure irritates a few people who are refused transport, but the rescue unit is immediately freed and available for the next call. This rapid return of the unit to a ready status enables the rescue ambulance service to operate with fewer units than would be possible if all patients were transported without question. It also lightens the load on the emergency departments by sorting out nonemergency cases and deters calls from people merely wanting transportation to a hospital for routine appointments or nonemergency conditions. The primary drawbacks to such a system are the political pressures to transport everyone in a city-operated system and the natural urge to transport all who can pay in a commercial-ambulance system.

Field treatment cases initially fall into categories of trauma (33%), illness (36%), respiratory and cardiovascular (21%), and other (10%). The effectiveness with which these can be treated in the field vary with the category.[4]

Trauma

Trauma treatment is generally confined to the visible manifestations and is relatively simple in the field environment, although omission of basic procedures can lead to death. In trauma, the EMT must insure an airway, check bleeding, occasionally maintain circulation, immobilize, treat for shock (including I-V when indicated), and extricate carefully. Further treatment must be given in a hospital; this treatment is frequently critical in such injuries.

Treatment of general illnesses varies greatly with the type but reassurance and careful handling are common denominators.

Coronary Care

Possibly the greatest challenge in field treatment is the coronary patient, always highly susceptible to sudden cardiac arrest. With the advent of cardiopulmonary resuscitation, portable DC defibrillators, and newer cardiac drugs, the trained EMT, assisted by other team members, can render treatment well beyond the capability of a physician only a generation ago and sometimes impossible for a physician working alone today. Cardiovascular disease kills more persons yearly in this country than all other causes combined.

Although the EMT will see only one heart attack for every three trauma cases, he should realize that the heart attack is 25 times as deadly as the injury. Not only is the high fatality rate a dramatic factor, but time is an ever present consideration in dealing with the coronary patient: of those who die of myocardial infarction, over half die in the field before reaching hospital medical care.

Because of the complexity of treatment covering a wide spectrum of heart and vascular disease as well as other physical conditions that may mimic heart disease, radioed medical advice from well-qualified physicians is required, especially if drugs are to be administered. To intelligently order treatment, the physician must be given a rapid but complete picture of the patient's condition, including history, vital signs, and impression of ECG readout, or preferably a telemetered ECG. In case of extreme emergency or loss of radio contact, the EMT should have prewritten orders. The execution of either radioed or pre-written orders requires a high degree of training and ability to operate under pressure.

Development of Field Treatment

Field treatment by the EMT following radioed advice is in reality an evolutionary process. Though speeded up to a great extent by the experience of three major wars and the virtual disappearance of the physician from the field environment, it is well to remember that treatment by medical corpsmen under radioed guidance by physicians ashore or on other ships has been accepted practice at sea for a half century. The advent of the highly trained EMT rendering relatively sophisticated medical treatment in the civilian community reflects the application of military combat medical technology to the civilian population. Its feasibility is rarely questioned today by medical professionals who have dealt with the problem firsthand. It is essential to remember that the comparison is not between the quality of care rendered by a physician and an EMT; the comparison is between the quality of care rendered by an EMT (backed by a physician) and no care at all!

TRANSPORTATION TO THE HOSPITAL

High-speed emergency runs to the hospital are seldom necessary if the patient is properly stabilized at the scene and in fact are detrimental to patients with certain classes of injuries or illnesses. With the acknowl-edged rougher ride of the more modern ambulances, it is even more important that patients with fractures or painful trauma be properly immobilized and transported carefully at moderate speeds. One common exception is severe internal trauma with hemorrhaging requiring surgical intervention; another is poison ingestion and overdose.

Patients should be strapped in and secured as much as is practical, and the attending EMT should be in a secure seat while not actually working on the patient. The numerous instruments and projections in the medical cabin of the ambulance make it a hazardous place to be thrown in a collision.

Hospitals should always be advised when a patient is en route. When the patient is not in critical condition, this information can be radioed into the control center and passed from the center to the hospital by telephone. When transporting a critical patient, the ambulance attendants should contact the hospital direct by radio, advising the type of case, brief history, vital signs, patient's doctor, and time of arrival. When transporting a heart patient, an ECG should be telemetered, and if resuscitation is in progress, the hospital cardiac resuscitation team should immediately prepare for the patient's arrival.

En route, the hospital can monitor the ECG and prescribe further treatment or medication if indicated. As a matter of economy, only one or two hospitals in an area need have ECG telemetry capability and can monitor a patient en route to it or any other hospital. All hospitals should have two-way voice radio communications with the ambulance, with control, and with each other and may give medical advice when required.

Normally, one EMT in the back with the patient will be sufficient. With critical patients, especially those under cardiopulmonary resuscitation, several men may be needed. As most emergency ambulances can only economically provide two persons, the additional men must be obtained at the scene from other sources. Police and fire fighters are the ideal source for the added manpower needed to handle the patient and administer team treatment. In Jacksonville, Florida, two EMTs ride in the back with any patient under cardiopulmonary resuscitation and are assisted by one fire fighter, providing a three-man team. The unit is driven by a fourth man, a fire fighter drafted from the fire company at the scene. The fire company will follow the ambulance to the hospital and pick up the two fire fighters after the patient is delivered. This system is the most cost-effective yet developed to provide the added trained manpower when needed.

TURNOVER AT THE HOSPITAL

The hospital, having been notified in advance of an incoming patient, should be appropriately prepared. While the lesser emergency may have to wait a reasonable time, there is no excuse for not being prepared for a critical case. If the hospital cannot be ready owing to circumstances beyond its control, the ambulance and patient should be diverted to another hospital with a higher readiness condition. As a rule, patients are carried to the hospital of their or their doctors' choice; all rescue ambulance crews should have "override" authority, however, to divert to another hospital should the patient's condition worsen dangerously or the original destination hospital be unprepared to receive the patient. If a hospital is to represent itself to the public as a first-line provider of emergency care, it must be able to provide quality care around the clock.

On arrival at the hospital with a critical case, the rescue crew has a right to expect members of the emergency department team on the platform to assist in moving the patient into the emergency department area without interruption of treatment. Even a minute's interruption in cardiopulmonary resuscitation during the turnover can result in irreversible damage, while an unnecessary delay in beginning hospital treatment can have grave effects on the outcome of a critical case.

The hospitals in a community will find it mandatory to increase the level and quality of emergency care as the field treatment and ambulance subsystems improve. The patient who would have been dead on arrival under a poor field treatment subsystem will arrive at the hospital as a critical patient when handled by a sophisticated rescue system. The hospital must be prepared to deal with this change in pattern; failure to do so will result in public criticism being shifted from inadequate field treatment by ambulance personnel to the failure of the hospital emergency department and physicians.

AIR TRANSPORTATION

A helicopter, though a highly effective transportation vehicle, is similar to an ambulance in that it is merely a component of the transportation subsystem to the EMC system. With good road systems, a ground ambulance can usually move a patient as rapidly as a helicopter within a radius of 35–50 miles. Beyond that, the helicopter is more effective in terms of time. Beyond 100–150 miles, the fixed-wing aircraft is more effective than either the helicopter or the ambulance, provided landing fields or strips are available.

If a well-developed ground ambulance system exists, there is relatively little requirement for helicopters. In thinly populated areas, however, and population centers located long distances from major medical centers, economic factors and time/distance considerations may preclude the establishment of an adequate ground ambulance system, and air transportation may be operationally desirable.

The helicopter is more costly to operate than a fixed-wing aircraft, which in turn is more costly than a ground ambulance. In view of this high cost and the relatively few cases that require aerial transport over an intermediate distance, few areas of the United States can afford helicopters for medical transport alone. This finding has been proved in a number of demonstration projects; there are some exceptions.

One exception is when the helicopter is used primarily for other missions, such as law enforcement, but can be diverted on a priority basis for medical evacuations. This system has proved highly successful with the Maryland State Police helicopters. Maryland is a small state, however, having three helicopters well-dispersed for normal patrol operations and a specialized and outstanding trauma research center ready to receive patients at a geographic location near the center of the state. The transport cases are mostly confined to trauma, and working space inside the small helicopters is not as critical as it would be with a cardiac arrest victim.

Another exception involves the use of military helicopters under the MAST program, by the Search and Rescue forces, or by special local arrangement with a military command. These helicopters are primarily used for military missions but can be made available for civilian medical emergencies on request. They are generally large enough to handle any type of case and do not require funding by the civilian community. Crews are not always available immediately, however, and long delays can result, which will more than nullify the speed advantage of the helicopter. The shortage of hospital corpsmen and doctors in the military and some reluctance by the military to risk possible liability in civilian cases are perhaps even more serious. So acute is this personnel shortage that some city EMC systems such as Jacksonville have agreed to provide the medical crews if the military will provide the helicopter and flight crews. While the time elements involved have made the use of the helicopter questionable within a 50-mile radius, we should also consider that an ambulance will be far better provided with equipment and medical supplies than will a helicopter, for which the equipment must be loaded on each mission.

Fixed-wing aircraft are much more commonly used than helicopters, primarily by charter or private ambulance companies for transfer of patients over relatively long distances between hospitals. The medical air evacuation system of the United States Air Force Military Airlift Command is frequently made available for transport of civilians in the national and humanitarian interest. Burn patients are frequently evacuated to Shrine burn hospitals by this method, and the Shrine is prepared to coordinate such missions with the military.

Written or taped records should be complete enough both to allow reconstruction of the case when necessary for critique and to accumulate data required for systems analysis, management, and budget purposes.

Record-keeping should start in the EOC. Cards should be time-punched to show the time of alert, dispatch, arrival on scene, at the hospital, and back in service. Twenty-four-hour tapes should record all radio and telephone conversations in order to obtain replays of events and provide legal protection.

A record of events in the field should be kept by the EMT in charge of the ambulance. For an organization with a heavy volume of calls, such a report should be designed for automatic data processing. Multiple carbon copies will make it possible to distribute one report to a number of locations, such as the ambulance headquarters, the accounting section for billing, with the patient as he is taken into the hospital, etc. This report, with the time punch card, should have enough data to allow a real time reconstruction of all events from alert to completion, including all patient data and treatment details, as well as difficulties encountered and remarks.

The emergency department record should cover events from entry until the patient is processed out of the emergency department. A cross-reference numbering system should allow a correlation of ambulance, emergency department, and hospital records.

The end results should be a weekly or monthly statistical summary of operations; a case by case summary of all individual cases; and individual summaries of specific desired data, all by means of automatic data processing. Weekly death audits may prove helpful in bringing out discrepancies, as will postmortem results of selected cases.

The purpose of all records is to establish what is taking place so that effective command and control can be exercised and performance optimized. If any record does not contribute toward this end, its continuation should be challenged.

REFERENCES

[1] Ambulance design criteria. National Academy of Engineering, Washington, U.S. Government Printing Office, 1971

[2] Essential equipment for ambulances. Bull Am Coll Surg 55:7–13, 1970

[3] Garrett CW: Which type of ambulance. Em Med Serv 2 (4), p. 11

[4] Jacksonville Fire Division. Official records, 1974

[5] Medical requirements for ambulance design and equipment. U.S. Department of Public Health. Publication No. (HSM) 73–2035, Washington, U.S. Government Printing Office, 1973

Donald G. Penterman

7

Telecommunications

Communications is that very vital link required for rapidly obtaining professional medical services or professional medical advice. This link and the wise management of all resources can well mean life or death for the critically ill or injured person. Many lives could be saved and much disability prevented simply by the prompt, systematic application of already established principles of emergency medical care. The problem is usually one of time and distance.

As noted in previous chapters, an emergency services system should provide quality care to any patient in the shortest possible time anyplace. Establishing communication links, properly systematized and managed in a manner to provide immediate action for emergency medical services (EMS), is the challenge faced in providing an effective telecommunications system *(the hands with knowledge, or the knowledge sent to other hands).* Bringing the Far, Near. . . . Now!

THE REGIONAL COMMUNICATION CENTER

An Interface for Systems

The essential requirement in designing a communications system is to provide an interface capability for all mobile radio and telephone systems operating within the region being served. Such interface location will not only allow existing and planned radio networks of all public service agencies to be linked together for relayed voice but, when desired, can also provide the capability for direct cross-talk between mobile units operating on different radio frequencies (channels) as well as direct connections to the existing telephone system (commonly known as radio-phone patching). The center can accommodate the phase-in of modern technology, while allowing continued use of existing older equipment and systems of separate agencies.

The importance of providing an interface communication center is being pushed by new designs in manufactured equipment, and EMS radio frequency changes are being brought about by the Federal Communication Commission (FCC). These FCC frequency allocations and rules should be carefully screened to allow the proper interface to telephone and radio systems to be designed into the communication center. The term "emergency use" is of utmost importance when reviewing FCC operational rules and procedures.

With a regional center for interconnect of systems (interface), all circuits and means of telecommunications (voice, print, or picture) can then be properly meshed for separate agency day-to-day use and be on ready standby for any type of emergency requiring linked communication for a team response with resources of multiple agencies.

Public and private services frequently cross jurisdictional boundaries when moving to meet the needs of an urgent call for assistance. Properly managed centers can immediately identify and overcome any jurisdictional problem, putting EMS needs as top priority.

Research continues to extend telecommunication technology, while seeking new applications of currently available technologic developments. Research to meet the needs of our space programs has excited and expanded technology. No telephone system existed on the moon, yet man's medical condition was continually monitored, discussed, and documented. Examples of these advances in technology are evident in the areas of the microwave market expansion (point-to-point air-wave circuits); growth in broad-band cable communications networks and application of a wide range of educational electronic systems and equipment; new telecommunications applications to oceanographic, space, law enforcement, highway, and medical systems; an increasing use of lasers; and an expanded use of integrated circuits and other solid-state circuitry. Voice or picture, printed or written words can now be provided at any location, mobile or fixed.

The United States Senate, in the course of considering the Emergency Medical Services Systems Act of 1973, stated that

> An emergency medical services system shall . . . join the personnel, facilities, and equipment of the system by a central communications system, so that requests for emergency health care services will be handled by a communications facility which: (1) utilizes emergency medical telephone screening; (2) utilizes, or, within such period as the secretary prescribes, will utilize the universal emergency telephone number 911; and (3) will have direct communication connections and interconnections with the personnel, facilities, and equipment of the system, and with other appropriate emergency medical services systems.[1]

Clearly, this is a recognition that telecommunications has an important role in the provision of emergency health care and medical services.

Technology to provide quality care in emergency medical services and rural health care already exists. The problem is one of organization to use this technology effectively and efficiently.

EMS SYSTEM DESIGN

The implementation of a telecommunication system assumes the ultimate existence of a response system, with action directed toward providing required, prompt, effective help via a multi-agency coordinated team effort.

Both systems, telecommunications and response, must be implemented to pull the subsystems together. The effectiveness of this pull-together action is based entirely upon the community, area, or region-oriented initiative and desire. Until a totally coordinated response system is installed (*i.e.*, fire, medical, police, public safety, utilities, sheriff, etc.) and the need to coordinate actions occurs, the primary reason for a consolidated telecommunication system does not exist.

Disaster reports continually emphasize that the weakness in service is in prompt creation of a team effort—a multi-agency coordinated response.

A telecommunication system designed to meet disaster needs, for which multi-agency coordinated action is essential to prompt assistance as well as critical conservation of resources, can greatly enhance the regular day-to-day operation of all involved agencies. Additionally, day-to-day usage assures workability in times of disaster.

Planners must define the plan of operation for use for all EMS resources (mobile and fixed units), before designing the communication system with links to and between these resources (Fig. 7.1).

Most of us are aware that an EMS system involves such obvious resource components as hospitals, medical clinics, ambulances, doctors, and nurses. Yet, these resources are only some of the essential parts required in an emergency medical services system. A truly effective EMS system, with full-service intent, includes not only medical elements but also all public service manpower and machines (fixed and mobile), administratively structured to provide the operational framework under which the coordinated and cost-effective management of all resources can be promptly accomplished.

A system denotes teamwork, with all subsystems working smoothly together as efficiently managed resources. The personnel of these subsystems must be qualified to perform as a member of the system. Training of personnel, individually and in team-action positions, becomes an essential requirement in an effective system. This training includes medical training for service dispatchers (resource managers) and public service agencies, as well as communications system training for all medical and paramedical staffs and personnel of all components of the total system, public service agencies, *i.e.*, police, fire, and utilities.

The levels of treatment available in the region—the life-support capability of each resource (man and/or machine); the education of the public; the demographic characteristics of the population served; terrain characteristics; weather problems; the interactions necessary for prompt, quality service—are all parts to be considered, evaluated, and linked by decisions of a common council, with singleness of purpose—*save lives, reduce disability and suffering!* The telecommunication system is but a tool, a very vital tool!

EMS TELECOMMUNICATIONS: THE PRIMARY OBJECTIVE

The primary objective of the telecommunications subsystem is to provide the necessary links to minimize the lapse of time between the life-threatening or crippling incident and the rendering of medical service. Response time formulas or goals have not been determined with any degree of validity. Yet it is important that a goal for response time can be established in each region being served by a planned EMS

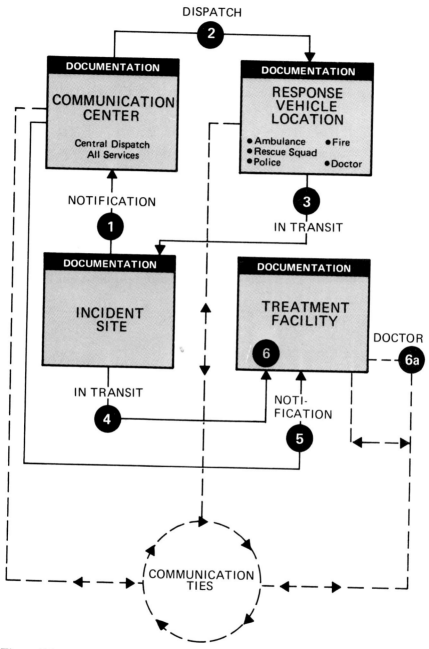

Figure 7.1
Plan of operation of emergency medical service resources.

system. With communications in full alignment, possibly two goals should be considered, setting acceptable limits for (1) receiving of on-scene advice and (2) arrival on-scene of trained personnel.

The medical profession widely recognizes that the provision of adequate treatment within 1 hour following a heart attack or other serious incident will more often than not determine whether the victim will live or die or be permanently disabled. Apparently, little study has been accomplished as to sustaining life until help arrives via remote advice to the scene.

Effective telecommunications can substantially minimize the time lapse between emergency incident occurrence at sites remote from treatment facilities and the rendering of treatment. Planners need to consider how existing telecommunications, in a defined operational region, can be interfaced, interconnected, integrated, and/or expanded, rearranged, or modified to meet the requirements of the EMS system. Most communities and local governments have a multiplicity of telecommunications services, facilities, and systems already available that relate in varying degrees to the mission of the EMS telecommunications subsystem. Yet, these many systems have not been interconnected in a manner to allow full use of existing circuits or equipment capability.

THE EMS SYSTEM TO BE SERVED BY TELECOMMUNICATIONS

Emergency medical services is evolving as a system—a new coordinated field of specialized professional medical services being organized to serve the sequence of actions surrounding a medical emergency wherever it may be located.

The basic elements of a full system (Fig 7.2) consist of (1) notification (the public call for help); (2) communication center (receipt of "help" call, dispatch of service response units, coordination of team action, alerting of facilities and medical professionals for support of action being directed); (3) response and transport units (ambulance, rescue, police, fire, mobile cardiac, poison, neonatal, etc.); and (4) fixed facility for life care (hospital, trauma clinic, special care units, doctor's office, etc.).

Notification

The public telephone system is the primary means used in "start action-call for help." To assist in reducing the time lapse between occurrence

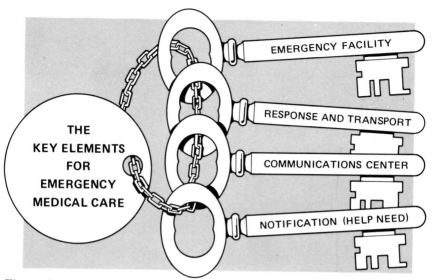

Figure 7.2
Key elements for an emergency medical care system.

of an incident requiring EMS and the rendering of services, a national common emergency telephone number, 911, is being encouraged and established, including a special feature of "no coin required" for pay-station telephones. Substantial progress has been made nationwide in this movement to assist in expediting the call for aid, which is often required under very emotional conditions.

Since the time frame for "service needed" begins when the incident occurs, the public automatically becomes a part of the EMS system, and public education on "how and what to report" to the regional communication center can assist in conservation of time. Responding with proper resources to handle the need is initially based on public identification of required assistance.

Establishing a 911 system for a community dictates consideration of a regional approach for a communication center (911 center), since the telephone exchange (circuits) boundaries do not coincide with medical service jurisdictional boundaries.

The implementation of a 911 system by the telephone industry can only be accomplished when the political jurisdiction decides where calls are to be answered on a 24-hour basis (Fig. 7.3). This 911 call-in establishes the first need for the center for the interface of a regional telecommunication systems. The call from the public starts the action

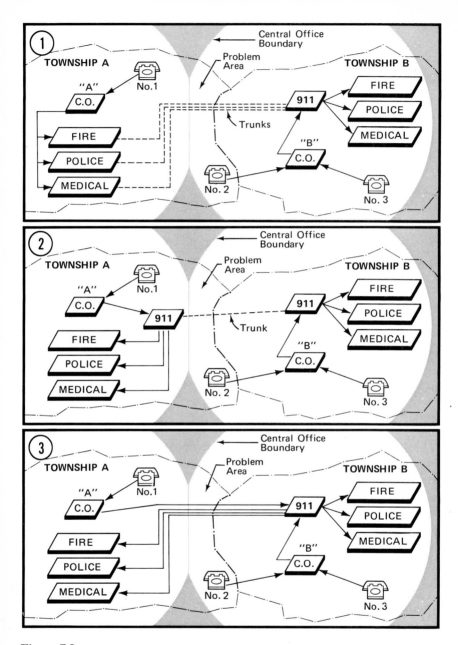

Figure 7.3
Methods for handling 911 calls when they go across emergency agency's jurisdictional boundaries. 1, 2, and 3 are representative of problem situations. Each situation has two adjacent communities: townships A and B.

requirement for a coordinated response with proper resources. A 911 system assumes a response system (Fig. 7.4).

Telephone company officials should be included in much of the organizational planning, since they can offer assistance and advice in service configuration. Once the system is in operation, it is the responsibility of the communication center director or other persons in governmental authority to handle the organization of the center. The telephone company will, of course, handle all maintenance of equipment provided by the telephone company and lines for the center.

The telephone company usually pays for the equipment additions and rearrangements in central offices necessary to accommodate the 911 number, including required changes for coin-free pay telephones. The community or region getting the 911 system pays for trunk lines from telephone central exchanges to communication center, lines from the center of the various jurisdictional agencies, and any telephone equipment needed at the communication center and its operation.

There are other service features that could enhance the 911 system that are available in some areas. One is "hold" and "re-ring." This service allows the 911 operator to call back a 911 caller to get further information about an emergency. This is especially helpful when dealing with children or excited callers who forgot to give the location of the emergency or other necessary information. Hold and re-ring also allows a 911 operator to trace bomb threats or false alarms.

Another auxiliary service is forcible disconnect. This service allows the 911 operator to disconnect a nonemergency call that is tying up the 911 line.

Even though these services enhance a 911 system, they are by no means necessary to the implementation of the system. The opening of the regional communication center lends itself to accepting calls from existing public mobile radio systems, thereby spreading the capability to mobile reporting or notification for the call for assistance. Additionally, on-street fire alarms and roadside emergency call boxes can be directly connected and the public encouraged to use them. With coin-free 911 calling at the telephone pay stations, these additions can substantially enhance the notification capability of the mobile public.

Citizen band radio emergency frequencies, keyed at the communication center, can assist in rapid reporting of accidents if properly organized. Actions can be taken to further broaden the mobile notification capability by accommodating radio frequencies by direct means or telephone circuits to other agencies or services having mobile radio systems in use, i.e., taxis, truckers, utilities, bus lines, school buses, wrecker service, etc.

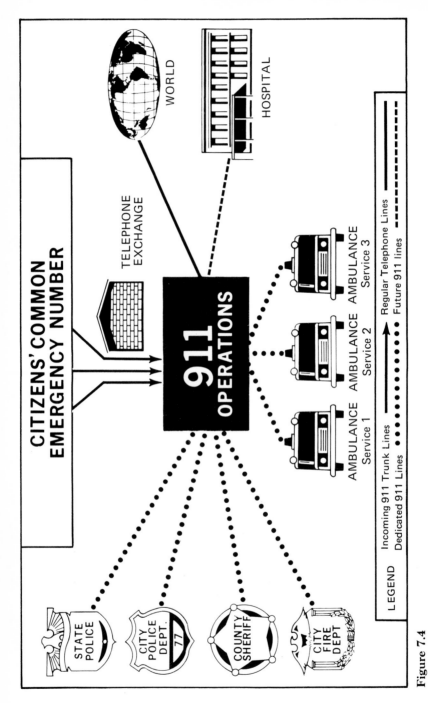

Figure 7.4
Operation of the 911 telecommunication system.

Summarizing notification (the public tie). (1) standard emergency telephone number 911; (2) citizen band mobile radio reporting; (3) public education; and (4) other mobile radio-equipped units (organized for eyes on the road reporting).

The Communication Center

The purpose of the communication center is for the interface of radio and telephone circuits and the management of all emergency resources responding to the usual myriad of day-to-day emergencies involving many people and a vast variety of emergency service needs.

These day-to-day needs are usually randomly spaced and generally involve limited numbers of people. A major disaster is identified by the immediate volume of services required and persons affected. In both cases the same EMS resources are involved. Experience has shown that a more effective coordinated service response can best be met through operation of an area-wide (regional) emergency communication center, where the direction and control of all resources can be effectively managed, supported, and supplemented as the degree of damage or threat to life may require. A properly coordinated response to. day-to-day emergencies can exercise procedures planned for handling a major disaster. An EMS system is one essential part of the disaster response system of a community, region, or area.

The purpose of the center is to operate 24 hours a day, 7 days a week for resources management by coordinating information from all major segments of city services, such as police, fire, medical, sanitation, and other essential resources, and shall serve as a municipal command center during enemy attacks, riots, daily emergencies, and naturally occurring disasters, such as earthquakes, major fires, snowstorms, tornados, and hurricanes.

The center should also coordinate its information for use by the municipal decision maker on a preventive basis. By gathering and assimilating the available information, city authorities can recognize trends toward emergency situations and thereby take action to avert an emergency rather than merely taking action after the emergency occurs.

It must, however, be recognized that the effective utilization of available EMS resources (all hospital, ambulance, rescue, mobile intensive care, etc., in the system) can best be accomplished through a central communications system for management and control. In most cases, co-location with another emergency service, or operated as part of a total community emergency operation center, is operationally beneficial and economically desirable. As daily operations of the EMS system are observed, one begins to see volume benefits from a co-location of a central 911 center (the interface with the public) and all emergency resources managed from a single location, sectioned to meet any special requirements of an individual service function.

Some community-wide or regional systems may require only one resource management (dispatch) center, including EMS, on the basis of the volume of emergency calls. Others, possibly large metropolitan areas, may need several centers, always with communication ties and common system radio service to assure intraregion service coordination and compatibility (Fig. 7.5).

The dispatching of medical aid involves ambulances, rescue units, and qualified medical personnel as required. It can include police, fire, public utility, tow trucks, and other units. At times of major disasters, heavy construction equipment, food, shelter, and other extraordinary services may also be required.

Standard dispatching technique should require that the driver of the responding vehicle notify the dispatcher of the time of departure to the scene, arrival at the scene, departure from the scene, delays encountered en route, arrival at a hospital, and readiness for another assignment. The times of these actions should be recorded to permit an analysis of the system-response effectiveness and for protection against claims of avoidable delay.

In addition to the initial dispatch, the dispatcher should be able to provide routing information to vehicles in transit, specifying the quickest route from the standpoint of distance, road conditions, and congestion. The dispatcher also must be able to call ancillary aid from other agencies. Thus, he requires direct-communication links with the bases where ambulances are deployed, with all vehicles by means of two-way voice radio, with all hospitals in the system, and with the emergency response dispatchers of other services, such as police, fire, public utilities.

Many patients die unnecessarily on the way to the hospital, when the use of proper stabilization techniques employed at the scene and during transit might have saved their lives. The effectiveness of such techniques, practiced by well-trained and well-equipped emergency medical technicians on board the ambulance with physician direction by means of two-way voice radio, has been well documented; yet few communities in the country have such systems at this time.

Of utmost importance in all of this action is documentation by tape and memo, covering service actions and medical advice given. Advice that is given is based upon information received, evaluated, and analyzed.

The requirement is clear: Central coordination of the response to a

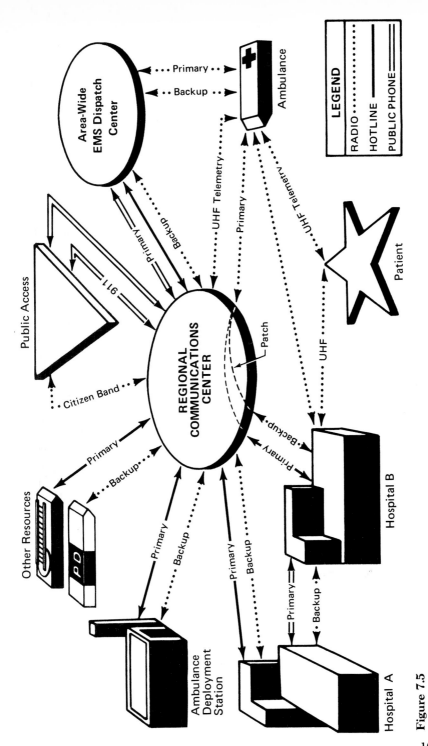

Figure 7.5
Model regional emergency communication system.

109

medical emergency, including the central dispatching of all emergency ambulances and other rescue units, and single-point coordination with other agencies are essential to an area-wide EMS system.

The communication center then accommodates the interface for umbrella communication coverage of the area, utilizing all mobile radio and telephone systems.

Within the area, the center can then provide immediate

Cross-talk capability between radio frequencies;
Radio to telephone interconnects;
Full-monitor or control capability of all agency radio calls when required;
Base radio-station individual or "all-call" capability to all radio-equipped mobiles;
Hand-carried radio units (portable) used "out-of-car" and in touch over the entire area or even long distances with other compatible areas with radio to telephone connections;
Connections to all commercial and public telephone service;
Full flexibility of circuit use to minimize and even eliminate busy signals;
Cross-talk capability created between mobile and fixed-point radio units of all agencies;
Select-call capability by digital dial for mobile to mobile or mobile to point;
Use of existing radio frequencies as allowed while phasing into FCC required changes;
Digital entry message devices, circuits for telemetry and facimily properly administered to obtain maximum use, reducing idle line time;
Manual or automatic recording of all actions;
Use of the public telephone number 911;
Standby electric power.

Summarizing the communication center. The center provides (1) 24-hour answering service to the public, along with service for and between all resources; (2) trained center operators with emphasis on medical terminology; (3) interface of all radio and telephone systems; (4) prompt connections to all hospitals, doctors, ambulances, and other resources by backup communications if required; and (5) citizen band radio service for the public assistance needs.

Transport and Hospital Telecommunications

Basic requirements. The basic requirement for the establishment of an EMS radio communication system between ambulance, hospital, and the regional communication center must take into account the existing systems and practices, as well as providing for the inclusion of all EMS vehicles into a common system. Provision must be made for the interfacing of the existing systems as well as the transition of the existing mobile systems into what might be termed a common system.

A common system: multi-channel capability. A common system means the use of multiple radio channels (frequencies) within the vehicle and within the emergency department of the hospital. In order to visualize the conveniences and simplicity of multiple radio channel hardware, it might be likened to multiple lines on a push-button, select-line telephone instrument. Like telephone instruments, radio units have their individual-call capability by numerical coding, and they provide for an all or selected group-call capability as desired by system planners. This multiple line arrangement provides maximum use of circuits and full flexibility for grouping emergency resources in a manner to allow cross-talk for coordination of action for a specific incident. Simultaneous incidents can then be managed on separate channels with no interference or allow for push-button line service if cross-channel interconnection is required. A "channel guard" on radio units can provide full monitoring of all channels when desired.

The communication center, as the dispatch and resource management center, should establish standard procedures for channel use and provide coordination of channel assignment during moments of high action when more circuits may be required. Achievement of the required level of efficiency in channel utilization will depend on channel time-use consideration and control.

Planners of the EMS system are starting to recognize the great flexibility that this common system approach can provide, although implementation to establish this common system becomes rather difficult in areas where available frequencies are already in heavy use. Some planners fail to acknowledge the importance of this task and take the easy solution of adding more equipment to one frequency (more on channel equipment; thus more clutter when heavy traffic occurs). Multiple channels can expand line capability manyfold, as a controller or automatic selector can utilize any open channel. By planned grouping of local government frequencies, many places can readily accommodate this approach and properly phase into a common system as new multi-channel radio equipment is procured.

To realize the full value from the multi-channel concept, all EMS vehicles and hospitals should be equipped with the capability of selecting any of the open channels, although normal use may allocate a primary-use channel to each ambulance or hospital.

111

As noted in the preceding section on the communication center, the common system approach can provide for a cost-effective interface for existing radio systems to operate in a totally integrated system. When one examines existing radio hardware and requirements for ambulance to hospital communications in the light of the systems approach to EMS, then the problem becomes one of providing a communications system that will have basic features serving all EMS system elements. Additionally, there must be standards and procedures that provide the basis for operation in a common system.

Biomedical telemetry. There are those who feel that medical communications should be built around the use of telemetry—that vital body functions, submitted by telemetry from the incident location or from the moving vehicle to the hospital, are of top priority. Others believe that only voice is required for diagnosis and treatment. Most EMS system planners, however, acknowledge the need for voice in conjunction with telemetry, when telemetry is considered to be essential. Either requirement can be readily met in a planned multi-channel communication system.

Portable radio units. Portable radio units for voice or biomedical telemetry can be added to provide out-of-vehicle contact from the side of a patient either by relay through the ambulance radio or by direct contact with the hospital when distance and circuitry will allow.

As in-vehicle units, portable units with multiple channels can provide the hospital-based doctor with talk-back circuits for use while viewing vital body-sign signals being sent to the emergency department of the hospital. The time of occupancy of a radio channel will be related to the nature of an emergency and to the time required to treat and transport a victim to a hospital. If required, a dedicated channel can be available full time during an ambulance run—from the time of arrival at the scene until delivery at the hospital. The need for this hot-line channel will vary with the type and nature of an emergency.

The principal difference between the channels required for ambulance control and the channels required for medical coordination is the amount of time that a channel is used on each occasion. The ambulance control usually requires very brief contacts in each phase of the service action. Radio contact is generally made at the time the ambulance leaves on assignment, when the ambulance arrives at the scene, when it is ready to leave the scene, and when it is back in service after delivery of a victim to a hospital. Each of these transmissions should involve very brief occupancy of the channel. Thus, many ambulances and ambulance control points can share the same channel. There should be coordination for channel sharing in accordance with locally devised plans and procedures to make the most effective use of the available channels. For coordination of medical treatment, there will be a need for multiple channels to permit the simultaneous use of adjacent stations, so that no interference will occur during care.

The common system approach requires that all channels be available on a multi-channel basis, so that ambulance units may establish contact with and be contacted by the control stations at any time and any place, and appropriate channels may be immediately available to serve simultaneous needs in the same or adjacent areas (Fig. 7.6).

In addition to the requirement for a common means of communications to provide radio contact between an ambulance and the most appropriate nearby medical emergency facility, the transfer of a patient extending beyond the boundaries of a local system will require the in-vehicle radio to be capable of operating into other regions. Thus, it is very important to provide for the proper network and interconnection among local systems by long-distance point-to-point links that have the capability to extend the range of mobile radio communications. When the occasion demands, radio telephone interconnections can readily meet this need through communication interface.

The extent of the economic benefits that are possible with the common system approach may be appreciated by the fact that a fully equipped ambulance today may have as many as two or three radio units to satisfy the different EMS requirements. In a common system, all EMS communication functions will be possible in a single multi-channel equipment unit. In addition, the multi-channel structure of the common system will provide an economic means for achieving substantially improved availability of all channels for all purposes for all EMS elements.

Pagers for staffs of ambulance and hospital emergency departments. With tone codes assigned to pagers for identification, alert calls can be activated from the 24-hour communication center or other equipped locations. Economy and operational efficiency leans toward the regional communication center for location of push-button encoder. The activation of an alert can be for an individual, a group, or an all-call for emergency staffs.

The encoder automatically keys the radio transmitter. The pocket or location pager emits an audible tone, followed by voice message. Split-second channel use is required.

Summarizing response and transport (the mobile care). (1) 24-hour service; (2) radio communications (vehicle and portable) to hospitals

114

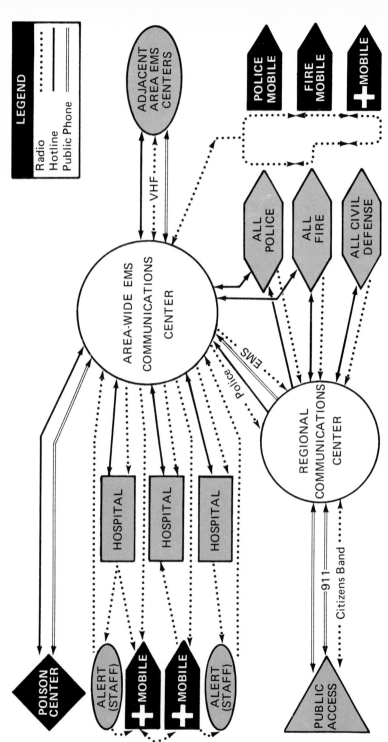

Figure 7.6
Model for area-wide emergency communication system.

and other mobiles; (3) telemetry (vehicle and portable); (4) hot-line radio to telephone connections; (5) trained EMT/A staffing (communication training); (6) radio coordination with special mobile intensive care or specialty units (poison, burns, hazardous chemicals, etc.); and (7) pagers for staff alerting.

Summarizing hospital emergency departments. (1) 24-hour service; (2) radio communications; (3) telemetry (where desired); (4) hot-line telephone-radio interconnect to all hospitals and mobile units; and (5) trained emergency department staff ("commo" training).

SYSTEM IMPLEMENTATION BY EVOLUTION

It is generally recognized that the effectiveness of day-to-day emergency medical operations depends greatly upon the provisions for assured and rapid communications, centralized dispatch, and coordination with all affected agencies. In general substance this means (1) area-wide radio and telephone communications for all hospitals and ambulances with select dialing capabilities; (2) area-wide and local paging (staff alerting); (3) central monitoring and resource coordination; (4) a common emergency telephone number for the public; and (5) capability for telemetry and hard-copy transmission.

The communications system as seen in Figure 7.6 should be established on a regional EMS basis to provide a comprehensive emergency medical service system, it being fully coordinated with or linked to the local governmental communications activities.

The evolutionary development of the EMS communication system will insure EMS of an early operational capability that can assist in providing answers for immediate service problems, while analysis and design activities continue on future phases of the system.

Problems in implementation and operation will also be somewhat minimized by the evolutionary approach. Some problems are associated with the evolutionary development, however. They often stem from the faulty assumption that succeeding phases for a region-wide system are independent and can be dealt with separately, when, in fact, each of the phases must be analyzed and designed with the objectives of the entire regional system at the forefront of the activity.

System planners should select the components to be included in each phase, based on decisions or such factors as cost, ease of implementation, and increased effectiveness.

REFERENCES

[1] Emergency Medical Services Systems Act of 1973. Report No. 93–397, Section 1206b, 93rd Congress 1st session, U.S. Senate, 1973

Don M. Benson
Maria Piantanida

8

Emergency Medical Technician Training

Historic breakthroughs in resuscitation and emergency care during the past two decades have made survival possible for people who in earlier years would have certainly succumbed to critical illness and/or injury. As experts from diverse fields study emergency care delivery systems, even more dramatic innovations can be expected. Because of this ever-growing technical knowledge, once cogent opinions, standards, and goals will be untenable. We, therefore, must recognize the need to periodically review our current medical practices against the new and higher opinions, standards, and goals engendered by exponentially accelerating growth of knowledge.

In developing EMS systems, as in all other areas of life, egocentrism (the state of thinking or acting with one's self as the major concern)[4]

117

plays a key role. As thinking people, we must not deny our own egocentrism. Instead we must recognize it as a primary motivating factor and critically consider what role our own personal and bureaucratic egocentrism plays in governing our response to new concepts.

These points should be intuitively obvious. Indeed, they should be part of the ethical code of all responsible health professionals. Thus many readers might interpret this apparently ludicrous sermonette as a blatant insult. The undeniable fact, however, is that individual and bureaucratic egocentrism has impeded progress in developing emergency care systems across this country and around the world. As a result, patients still asphyxiate unattended as they are rushed to the hospital at the highest possible speed. Victims of acute myocardial infarction still suffer ventricular fibrillation in the street without the opportunity for prompt defibrillation. People still exsanguinate from improperly applied tourniquets. People are still made quadraplegic from inexpert handling of unstable spine fractures. Bearing these thoughts in mind, we shall review the evolution of EMT training.

EVOLUTION OF EMERGENCY TRAINING

The concept of specialized training for ambulance and rescue personnel dates back centuries. In antiquity the Egyptians splinted fractures. More recently, Baron Dominique Jean Larrey, a Napoleonic army surgeon, devised light carriages for transporting soldiers from the battlefield. Personnel staffing Larrey's vehicles were trained in hemorrhage control and fracture splinting.[6]

The introduction of exhaled air ventilation (mouth-to-mouth/mouth-to-nose techniques) in the late 1950s and the reintroduction of cardiac compression in 1960 armed the emergency care provider with effective techniques for maintaining vital systems. For the first time the ambulance crew person could effectively intervene in the dying process.

The ensuing years brought improved methods for extricating from entrapment and for managing hypovolemic shock and acute myocardial infarction.

In 1966 the National Academy of Sciences/National Research Council Committee on Trauma in its now famous document, "Accidental Death and Disability: The Neglected Disease of Modern Society,"[9] called for improved training for ambulance personnel. In 1969 the Emergency Medical Services Committee of the National Academy of Sciences, National Research Council outlined the instruction deemed essential for ambulance and rescue personnel in the pamphlet, "Training of Ambulance Personnel and Others Responsible for Emergency

Care of the Sick and Injured at the Scene and During Transport."[10] Pursuant to this report, teaching aids including textbooks, slide sets, instructor lesson plans, and training manuals were developed by national and international organizations including the U.S. Department of Transportation,[2] the American College of Surgeons, the American Academy of Orthopedic Surgeons,[5] and the World Federation of Societies of Anesthesiologists.[8]

Perhaps most notable of these was the 81-hour training program for EMT-ambulance[2] published by the U.S. Department of Transportation in 1971. Subsequently, this suggested program evolved into a highly recommended guideline, then into an essential goal, and now a minimum standard enforced by threat of withholding federal funds from projects failing to comply. Although the 81-hour training program for EMT-ambulance has been a significant milestone, the rigidity with which the program can be enforced not only discourages but even prohibits introducing more efficient methods for accomplishing these same training goals. Curiously, the improved methods for accomplishing these same training goals have been developed largely on knowledge generated by conducting the 81-hour program.

For instance in 1971 a national conference on EMTs held in San Antonio, Texas, by the Academy of Orthopedic Surgeons recommended redesign of the basic 81-hour course to present complex psychomotor skills earlier in the course, revision of the requirements for admission to the course, and reexamination of the qualifications for instructors.[7] Regretably distribution of these recommendations has been very limited, and implementation has been virtually nonexistent.

In 1970 a task force of the National Research Council EMS committee convened to examine the training of advanced EMTs.[1] Based on the best information available, the task force recommended a 480-hour instructional program for training EMTs in definitive care skills. Since publication of these recommendations, thousands of basic EMTs have acquired the targeted definitive care skills in far less than 480 hours of instruction. Throughout the country, both professional and volunteer ambulance personnel have learned basic diagnostic electrocardiography, defibrillation, I-V infusion therapy, use of resuscitative and antiarrhythmic drugs, and endotracheal intubation in 100–150 hours of didactic sessions followed by supervised clinical and field experience.

While this knowledge was being accumulated, the U.S. Department of Transportation developed instructor lesson plans and instructional video tapes for the 480-hour advanced EMT training program. As of this writing, these instructor lesson plans are still being field tested. Thus the results of these experiences are not yet available.

BEHAVIORAL OBJECTIVES FOR TRAINING

As educational methodology experts began designing EMT training programs, the need to clearly define behavioral objectives for specific training courses was emphasized. Instructors and students can understand what is expected of them only after the behavior that the student is expected to display at the conclusion of the course has been described precisely and accurately. For instance, the statement "The EMT-basic must be able to secure a patent airway" is insufficient as a behavioral objective, for it leaves unclear such questions as "What types of airway obstruction [*e.g.*, hypopharyngeal soft tissue, foreign body] are present?" "In what types of patients [*e.g.*, unconscious, stuporous, conscious] does it exist?" "Should airway control techniques be limited to noncannulating methods?" and "If cannulating methods are used, should they include experimental techniques such as transtracheal jet injection?" Instead, the behavioral objective should read:

> The EMT-basic will be able to secure airway patency in the unconscious patient using the following noncannulating airway control techniques: hyperextension of the head, intermittent positive pressure ventilation—exhaled air technique, forward displacement of the mandible using the jaw lift and jaw pull maneuvers, removal of foreign bodies using the cross-finger maneuver and the oropharyngeal airway.

Even this behavioral objective is stated in terms so general that an instructor cannot accurately outline the lesson plan. The specific behavioral objective for the first component of the general objective given above might be stated as follows:

> The first noncannulating airway control step in the unconscious patient not suspected of having a cervical spine fracture is performed by simultaneously lifting the back of the patient's neck and pressing downward on the patient's forehead, the hand on the forehead being positioned so the nose can be grasped between the thumb and index fingers.

With behavioral objectives identified at general and specific levels, modular instruction can be developed allowing trainees to progress toward specific objectives at their own rate as determined by such factors as interest, ability, prior background, experience, and local community needs and resources.

Defining behavioral objectives is also a prerequisite for development of accurate, universally acceptable proficiency tests. Availability of such proficiency tests will allow identification of students who have satisfactorily achieved a given behavioral objective, thus permitting instructional resources required for attaining that objective to be devoted to another student.

Behavioral objectives for the basic and advanced EMT courses can provide solutions to many problems currently facing the field, including certification of personnel in multiple jurisdictions (*e.g.,* across state lines) and provision of nonredundant instruction for students with significant experience (*e.g.,* military corpsmen).

Developing behavioral objectives is a laborious task far beyond the scope of this chapter. Nonetheless, it remains an essential matter that must be addressed by appropriate agencies.

Training packages will be developed over the coming years. Some will adhere to the basic U.S. Department of Transportation standards; others will not.

The criteria for adequacy or inadequacy of these programs must not be their adherence to an antiquated standard or a newly established administrative regulation. Instead, their acceptability must be based on their ability to efficiently accomplish the desired objectives.

However laudable and rational the development of training programs based on sound behavioral objectives may appear, allotting instructional resources (instructors' time, teaching aides, classrooms, laboratories) requires some description of the number of instructional hours likely to be required for presenting a specific subject. A description of required clock hours is essential for budgeting time, salaries, space, and other resources, but we must recognize it as just that: as a statement of time required to present material. It is not a criterion of satisfactory course completion by the student.

CURRENT EMT SKILLS

In the present state of the art, most skills that EMTs can safely apply can be presented in a time frame of 200–230 hours (*i.e.,* 80 hours for the basic program and 120–150 hours for the advanced). These skills include basic and advanced life support; control of surface hemorrhage; splinting of spine and long bones; extrication from entrapment; use of medical command communications equipment, including biomedical telemetry equipment; and operation of emergency vehicles.

Emergency medical technicians wishing to enter related fields, such as industrial health and safety or ambulance service administration, might find other subjects (*e.g.,* group dynamics, teaching techniques, fiscal operation, and administrative management) useful. The behavioral objectives sought in these programs, however, are different from the patient-care objectives sought by EMT training. Thus, even though more extended instructional programs, such as the 2-year community college program, will produce personnel with highly desirable skills, these programs should include patient-care skills as one component and skills in related areas as a second, separate component. A 2-year program is not essential for those primarily interested in the basic and advanced life-support skills needed for patient care.

Endotracheal Intubation Training

Tracheal intubation is a skill that can be learned by EMTs without practice on live human patients. While carefully supervised practice on anesthetized patients under controlled conditions in the operating room is highly desirable, EMTs have learned the technique using carefully written protocols and guided supervision on intubation training manikins. In addition, some have observed intubation of the trachea in emergency departments and surgical theaters; and some have had a rare opportunity for cadaver practice. Both volunteer ambulance personnel (Shaler Township, Pennsylvania)[3] and full-time fire rescue personnel (Columbus, Ohio) trained by only these methods have successfully mastered the technique and proved their ability in field situations.

In conclusion, technologic advances of the past two decades have produced effective methods for intervening in the dying process. Properly trained, well supervised, highly motivated ambulance and rescue personnel can apply these methods in the field safely and effectively. The principle concern in developing training programs must revolve about the behaviors that students are to display at the end of the training program rather than the number of instructional hours the student logs. The conventional way of labeling programs in terms of clock-hours logged (81-hour course, 480-hour program, 2-year curriculum) diverts attention from the central issue of behavioral objectives to the secondary issue of the time required to present the material. Identifying time allocations required to present material is important for planning programs, but it must not supersede the main issue of proficiency.

Expanded knowledge, improved techniques, and development of new insights change recommendations and "standards." Therefore, all recommendations, including this one, must be critically reviewed periodically in the light of the current state of the art.

REFERENCES

[1] Advanced training program for emergency medical technicians—Ambulance. Washington, Division of Medical Sciences, Committee on Emergency Medical Services and the Subcommittee on Ambulance Services, National Academy of Sciences, National Research Council, 1970

[2] Basic training program for emergency medical technicians—Ambulance. Instructor's Lesson Plans. Washington, U.S. Department of Transportation, National Highway and Traffic Safety Administration, 1971

[3] Benson, DM, Weigel JA: Basic and advanced life support services by suburban volunteer fire departments (abstr). Annual Meeting of the American Public Health Association, San Francisco, November 4–8, 1973, p. 100

[4] Davies P (ed): American heritage dictionary of the English language. New York, Dell Publishing Co., Inc., 1969

[5] Emergency care and transportation of the sick and injured. Chicago, Committee on Injuries, American Academy of Orthopedic Surgeons, 1971

[6] Kennedy R (ed): Emergency care. Philadelphia, W. B. Saunders, 1966

[7] National Workshop of the Training of Emergency Medical Technicians. Recommendations and conclusions for an approach to an urgent problem. Committee on Injuries. Proceedings of Conference of the American Academy of Orthopedic Surgeons, San Antonio, July 22–23, 1971

[8] Safar P:Cardiopulmonary Resuscitation. A Manual for Physicians and Paramedical Instructors. World Federation of Societies of Anesthesiologists, 1968

[9] Seeley S (ed): Accidental death and disability: The neglected disease of modern society. Washington, National Academy of Sciences, National Research Council, 1968

[10] Training of ambulance personnel and others responsible for emergency care of the sick and injured at the scene during transportation. Washington, Committee on Emergency Medical Services, National Academy of Sciences, National Research Council, 1968

James D. Mills

9

Emergency Medical Technicians
Training and Salary

Most physicians and other viewers of the emergency medical scene will accept without documentation that competence of EMTs is directly related to their training. Observers know almost intuitively that readily available, well-trained EMTs do have a a very significant impact on the quality of emergency medical care and on the outcome of patients afflicted with trauma and illness.

Elsewhere in this volume, training opportunities, course content, and requirements are presented. The attractions encouraging men and women to choose EMS for a career and to remain in that career are background, job distinction, professionalism, salary, retirement benefits, opportunity for advancement, intellectual stimulation, and craftsman satisfaction.

In the job market generally, compensation is related to educational level as modified by the classical forces of supply and demand. Additional modifiers are political considerations, social economics, rewards for bodily risk, and rewards for unusual hours or days of work.

LEVELS OF TRAINING

The U.S. Department of Transportation has estimated that 250,000 people are involved in the delivery of medical transportation as drivers, mechanics, attendants, technicians, dispatchers, radio operators, and office personnel. Of these, over 50,000 have completed the Dunlap (Department of Transportation) 81-hour course. The National Registry of Emergency Medical Technicians has had 21,000 applicants for registration and has qualified 15,000 as registered EMTs.[3]

Emergency medical technicians may be considered as: (1) governmental, paid (almost always associated with police or fire departments; (2) volunteer, usually unpaid; and (3) private. Of those qualified as registered EMTs, the distribution is about equal in the three groups.[3]

Actual pay received by EMTs, whether trained or not, varies tremendously. For those without administrative duties, the range is from the legal minimum wage of $2.20 to $3.50 per hour. With the mandatory provisions requiring overtime pay and standby pay while on call, the annual income ranges from $3,300 to $14,028.

Since most governmental emergency medical transport services are under police or fire department supervision, the salaries of EMTs as well as their retirement benefits are hinged to those of police and fire fighters. They also have the opportunity to advance in the departmental hierarchy and in city governments.

When the operation is hospital based, the salary scale is related to that of the other hospital employees, the starting registered nurse salary serving as an effective ceiling for EMT starting compensation. In such a situation, EMTs look to the hospital milieu for their career advancement. In Tallahassee, Florida, a hospital-based ambulance service has seen several of its EMTs advance to physician. In Alexandria, Virginia, five EMTs in hospitals have received MD degrees or are pursuing that degree in medical school, and one former emergency technician is a dental student.

Students in biologic sciences who work part time and during school vacations are an excellent source for finding bright, strongly motivated EMTs.

From the medical point of view it seems desirable that municipal departments of public safety be divided into police, fire, and EMS. This division is not traditional, since the medical services have not reached the necessary level of complexity and political impact for such a degree of autonomy. It is recognized in some communities (such as in Middletown and Hamilton, Ohio; Los Angeles, California; Miami, Florida; and Houston, Texas) that EMTs trained also as fire fighters have additional skills and responsibilities, and they are provided with a salary supplement.

PRIVATE EMERGENCY CARE

In the private sector an ambulance company providing first-rate service in emergency care and also in ambulance transport must pay attractive wages and offer career advancement opportunities. It is probably fair to say that private companies are more sensitive to cost containment than those that are tax supported.

Such a company in the southeastern United States requires a high-school education, an 8-hour first-aid course from the American Red Cross, and the 81-hour Dunlap course for its beginning EMTs. It prefers men with military medical experience, and 95% of its EMTs have this background. The work is divided into 24-hour shifts of which 13 hours are work time, 8 hours are sleep time, and 3 hours are meal time. The starting pay is $3.19 per hour for the work and one and one-half times that amount for sleep or meal time interrupted by calls. With time off, these men clock in 52 and 39 hours in alternate weeks, their gross earnings being $310 every 2 weeks and their annual income $8,060 in 1974.

Salaries are step-graded with annual cost-of-living raises of 3.5–5% and annual merit raises of 2.5–5%. Representative advancement opportunities within the company are given in Table 9.1. Job descriptions in detail are presented by the Committee on Emergency Medical Services, National Academy of Sciences, National Research Council.

There is no retirement funding at present, but the recruitment of personnel does not seem to be hindered.

In this example an average EMT works in that position 2½ years and either advances within the business or moves on to other pursuits. Those going elsewhere find employment as hospital technicians, respiratory therapists, law enforcement officers, fire fighters, and EMT teachers. Some return to school to study political science, nursing, and medicine. They also advance to managerial positions in other private or in public ambulance systems.[6]

Those companies at the lowest range of compensation for ambulance attendants attract less-trained personnel and tend to be engaged in

Table 9.1. Advancement Opportunities

Title	Gross annual income range
Technicians	
EMT	$8,060–10,556
Assistant shift manager	8,892–12,402
Shift manager	9,802–12,402
Managers	
Training manager	11,336–14,820
Supplies manager	9,802–12,818
Assistant manager	9,802–14,820
Manager	14,456–18,928

ambulance transport. In these situations emergency medical transportation is done by others, either governmental or voluntary companies.

GOVERNMENTAL EMERGENCY CARE

In the interest of improving the total ambulance service of the United States, it would be useful to scrutinize the trend of dividing governmental service for emergencies and private service for transportation. The knowledge and skills that crews require to provide a high quality emergency ambulance service are also required to transport safely a seriously ill or injured person from one medical institution to another. The same standards of equipment and training should apply to all ambulance services licensed to transport the sick and injured.[4]

We are not encouraging the careers of paraprofessional EMTs when we require them to be fire fighters or policemen first, EMTs second. Emergency medical technicians should not owe their first loyalty and their opportunity for promotion to the fire or police department.

VOLUNTEER EMERGENCY CARE

Volunteer companies constitute about one-half of all those engaged in emergency medical transportation in the United States.[2] These men and women are motivated by public service and have a long and honorable history of performance. They are the backbone of rural service and serve as well in smaller cities and suburban counties. Generally they are not paid, although some jurisdictions do award stipends of the order of $5.00 for an ambulance call. Their rewards are the intangible ones of belonging to the group, often in a clublike atmosphere; the drama of the calling; civic duty; and the craftsman's satisfaction of performing a chosen calling well. Because with them it is an avocation and not their principal work, they expose themselves to the charge of dilettantism. Lured, perhaps, by the siren and flashing red light, many volunteers remain to become qualified as highly competent technicians.

Local innovations produced a modified volunteer rescue service in Killeen, Texas (population 42,000), which is adjacent to Fort Hood (40,-000 troops). Under fire department direction an ambulance service is operated with eight military medics actually assigned to that duty. The city bears the other costs of the operation, and the army pays the regular military salary to the EMTs. Service is provided to both military and civilian personnel.[5]

From afar, the prevailing view is that the best EMS care the people will receive is from a highly sophisticated and integrated nationwide EMS system. Until that day arrives we are grateful for the many volunteer companies who selflessly render service now.

EMT CAREERS

The career ladder for EMTs has many attractive rungs and future options. The stability of the system requires that a trained technician remains at his job long enough to justify his training. This requirement does not mean that once trained he is permanently locked in as an ambulance or hospital EMT. It may be, in fact, counterproductive for him not to seek advancement. The work is technical, to be sure; it requires high skill and training. It remains, however, a physical job as well, with physical demands that are less easily met with advancing age. Even with continuing education requirements, the senior EMT is less flexible and receptive to new ideas and techniques than juniors and is, therefore, liable to be less in demand unless protected by job tenure requirements.

As work satisfaction and prestige improve for EMTs, it is to be expected that these men and women will remain longer in their chosen fields. It follows that they will honor the implied commitment to improve their skills and keep abreast of new techniques.

In Alexandria, Virginia (a 120,000-population suburb of Washington, D.C.) all EMTs are qualified fire fighters. Once trained and then assigned to ambulance duty, they do not return to firefighting except on their own initiative. When serving as EMTs, they receive an annual supplement of $250. Beginning pay is $10,081 (plus the $250), rising to a theoretic $20,983 (plus $250) for an assistant chief with 14 years' service. In actual fact, the highest ranking EMT is a captain who earns $16,441 (plus $250) after 14 years' service. There are two lieutenants who earn $10,585 to $14,913 (each plus $250) after 14 years' service. This company is represented by a local of the American Federation of Labor-Congress of Industrial Organization in its negotiations with the city. Retirement begins at age 50 and pays 60% of the average of the 3 highest years' salary after 25 years of service. After 30 years of service the pension rises to 70%.

REPRESENTATIVE INCOMES

A survey in 1973 produced useful findings in demonstrating the range of compensation to be expected in the governmental managed companies of a dozen cities.[1] Omitted are detailed tenure and merit increases, the intent being to offer an overall idea of pay to be expected. All are within municipal or county fire departments except Boston, Massachusetts (police department), and Tallahassee, Florida (hospital based).

Baltimore: EMTs receive no supplement over the fire fighter's $8,700.
Boston: Policemen ride the ambulance units and receive the basic patrolman's salary of $16,640.
Columbus: Paramedics receive $12,000.
Dallas: EMTs (now designated paramedics) receive the same pay as fire fighters, $12,240. Advanced training has recently been instituted. Texas has legislation enabling paramedics to give drug and fluid therapy.
Houston: Fire fighters earn $9,300; EMTs, $10,200.
Jacksonville: EMTs earn $7,800; EMT lieutenants, $8,100.
Los Angeles city: The fire department administers an ambulance service that is in transition from a service made up of all fire fighters to one in which the personnel are not fire fighters. Ambulance drivers receive $12,564; ambulance attendants, $14,028. All are trained paramedics; some are from antecedent private companies in the area.
Los Angeles County: The fire department maintains a paramedic rescue service. Fire fighters receive $12,000; paramedics, $12,360.
Miami: Fire fighters receive $10,440; paramedics, $10,960. There are two paramedic lieutenants and one captain. One officer serves each 24-hour shift.
Tallahassee: County-wide hospital-based ambulance service. Basic EMTs receive $8,700. Paramedic training increases this base, and shift supervisors receive compensation pay.

Tampa: Within the fire department the basic fire fighter receives $9,-800; EMTs, $9,980. Each rescue unit comprises one EMT, one lieutenant, and one captain. Officers receive $180 per year supplement for this service.

Seattle: Fire fighters earn $10,500. Seattle has EMTs who receive a 10-cent hourly supplement and paramedics who receive a $900 annual supplement.

The business of providing skilled medical care at the site of the accidents and illness, while transporting the patients, and within the hospital is a very complex one. As a nation we tend to receive those services for which we are willing to pay. In professionalizing the EMT calling, we must refine our selection process and further formalize training requirements.

It is necessary to make use of the resources now at hand. Military medics, already in demand for physician's assistant careers, are an excellent resource. Community colleges stand ready to design and offer programs for EMTs. The U.S. Department of Transportation has made impressive accomplishments in course design. Emergency departments of hospitals can offer laboratory experience coordinated with formalized college programs.

However massive the national effort, trainees must have incentive in terms of prestige and reward to select the most capable potential.

REFERENCES

[1] Briese GL: personal communication

[2] Hulfish TH, McDade JP: Review, analysis, and alternatives of the ambulance situation in Alexandria, Virginia. Alexandria, Va., Paramed, Inc., 1971

[3] Morando RV: personal communication

[4] National Registry of Emergency Medical Technicians, Columbus, Ohio

[5] Rucher VB: GI's ride F.D. ambulances. Engineering, November, 1973

[6] Vestal WT: personal communication

III

Hospital Education
and Training

Milton N. Luria
John H. Morton

10

Education and Research in the Emergency Department

The hospital emergency department has always been an exciting place in which to work and to learn. In the past, faculties have been divided about the importance of this area in the education of medical students. Some clinicians have felt that the problems presenting in the emergency department can be too sensitive or too critical for active student participation and that the student's presence might slow the process of caring for the critically injured or sick. Others felt that the emergency department could not involve the student in a significant educational experience.

Since World War II, there has been a patient population explosion in emergency departments that has changed to a great extent the scope and the importance of the work in the emergency area. Much energy and money have gone into rethinking, reorganizing, and expanding the department to conform to modern day concepts of proper emergency care for the community and the hospital. The emergency department became an increasingly important institution for patient care in the 1950s and 1960s. Despite this, however, the teaching of emergency medical care still is given an insignificant role in the undergraduate and postgraduate programs of many medical schools. In the past few years, national organizations such as the University Association for Emergency Medical Services[3] and the American College of Emergency Physicians have attempted to stimulate interest in emergency training by developing and publishing guidelines for the education of medical students and residents in emergency medical services. The stated goals[2] of such programs are to prepare the physician to render care to the acutely ill or injured patient and to improve emergency medical care.

EDUCATIONAL OBJECTIVES OF THE UNDERGRADUATE TRAINING PROGRAM

There are several educational objectives that can be better achieved in an emergency department than elsewhere in the medical center. These goals became the cornerstone for a 4-week interdepartmental required Emergency Department Clerkship during the fourth year at the University of Rochester (New York) School of Medicine and Dentistry. During the student's emergency department experience he can come to understand and learn to deal with the following:

1. A portion of the disease spectrum which can be observed only in an emergency setting. This would include the acute phases of certain illnesses which require hospital admission, such as acute appendicitis, ruptured ectopic pregnancy, and acute cardiac arrhythmias, as well as certain common medical problems which are often managed in the emergency department without requiring hospital admission, such as acute streptococcal pharyngitis, uncomplicated pneumococcal pneumonia, acute hysteria, and Colles' fracture.

2. Patient problems which require rapid but accurate assessment. Traditionally, when the student is assigned to a patient during an inpatient clerkship, he takes a detailed medical history and carries out a meticulous physical examination. He may then supplement his knowledge by lengthy laboratory investigations before making a diagnosis and planning therapy. In an emergency department the student learns that this approach is not appropriate in all settings, and he receives training in making more rapid assessments. He also becomes aware of the pitfalls of such a technique and learns to differentiate a concise evaluation from a snap judgment. He should

also discover the benefits of a short period of observation in clarifying an uncertain diagnosis.

3. The proper disposition of a patient once the emergency has been managed. In deciding what should subsequently be done for the patient, the student becomes involved in arranging follow-up care and learns what services social agencies can contribute to community health.

4. The fact that the physician cannot always render medical care at a time of his own choosing. He should recognize that a problem which seems minor or even trivial to the physician may be important to the patient and that the patient's frame of reference must be appreciated.

5. The new role of the hospital as a source of primary care for many members of the community. He should also begin to appreciate the impact of the physician shortage.

6. The emotional reactions of patients and their families at a time of crisis.

7. Triage and its role both in the handling of large numbers of casualties and in maintaining the efficiency of the ordinary emergency department activities.[4]

During the 4-week emergency clerkship, the student rotates through the active services of the department, seeing a representative sample of both critical and nonurgent illnesses that present to the department. The student, under the supervision of a resident, takes the responsibility for evaluating the patient's problem, planning diagnostic studies, and further assisting in the therapeutic management of the patient. The student thus sees how the public and health-care professionals use an emergency department. He or she can develop an understanding of the broad scope of emergency treatment. The opportunity for the student to make the first medical contact with an acutely ill patient is intellectually stimulating and provides an important dimension to his acquisition of knowledge. In addition, the student is encouraged to follow his patients after they leave the emergency department either by admission to the hospital or by return appointment in the ambulatory-care area. The number of students assigned to any emergency service is small, allowing for close personal involvement and supervision of the student by the house staff. Daily seminars to permit general discussions of a whole range of emergency problems and bedside attending rounds to evaluate patients, particularly those being observed in the emergency overnight ward, allow the faculty to educate the students in a more formal manner.

To facilitate an active teaching program requires adequate conference room space within the emergency department. Audiovisual equipment and a modest library should be included in the plans for any emergency department with an active teaching program.

HOUSE STAFF TRAINING

The principles and goals enumerated above are equally applicable to the house staff working in the emergency department. Because of the way patients seek entrance to the health-care system and because of the way hospitals are organized, it seems inevitable that the acute phase or initial presentation of a broad spectrum of medical illness or trauma will be dealt with in the emergency department setting.

We believe that supervision and teaching of house officers in the emergency department is of vital importance. For years, residents have recognized the value of the practical experience gained working in this area. More frequently than not the experience was unsupervised, and no one was available to teach appropriate principles of emergency care or to correct bad habits. House officers are not allowed to work without supervision on an inpatient service. It is even more important to provide teaching and supervision in the emergency department.

There is still too little direct supervision of house staff activities in the emergency departments in this country. The experienced clinician possesses the knowledge and skill to care for the critically sick, but he has not been afforded the opportunity to share this knowledge with his junior colleagues. Instruction of house staff is the responsibility of senior attending physicians in the emergency department program at the University of Rochester. Experience in this program indicates that active attending teaching rounds are appropriate and that they need not slow or interfere with critical service functions. Indeed, formal teaching rounds have improved screening and expedited care in this critical area.

There are two types of instruction that may be organized in the emergency department.

Specialty emergency department.   The first type is for those hospitals in which the emergency department is organized according to specialties (*i.e.*, medicine, pediatrics, surgery, etc.). Each specialty should devote a significant part of its program to the emergencies encountered in that specialty. Faculty should be assigned to spend considerable time—if not full time—supervising and teaching the house staff about those critical problems unique to their specialty training. Thus the medical emergency or the surgical emergency gives another dimension to the instruction of the specialist in internal medicine or surgery.

Emergency physicians. The second type of instruction is for those emergency departments with full-time emergency physicians. Over the past decade a large number of emergency departments have employed full-time emergency physicians. These professionals have been recruited from the ranks of practicing physicians. Until recently, no doctors had been trained specifically to deal with the problems that are encountered in a busy emergency department. In the past 5 years, a number of medical centers have developed 2-year residency programs in emergency medicine to train physicians specifically for the role of this new specialty, the emergency department physician. This is an important development in emergency medical care. Since a number of hospitals are now employing full-time physicians to staff their emergency departments, these specialists must be adequately trained to fill a challenging new medical role.

OTHER EMERGENCY DEPARTMENT EDUCATION

There are other educational programs that should be organized by the emergency teaching staff. Programs of continuing education and postgraduate courses for practicing physicians—either traditional specialists or the new emergency department physicians—should be organized by the larger medical centers and national organizations devoted to emergency medical care. These programs should keep the physician abreast of the latest techniques and accepted practices in emergency work.[1] The emergency department of the University of Rochester offered in June 1974 for the first time an American College of Physicians postgraduate course: "Emergency Department Medicine for the Internist." We hope to repeat this course every few years.

Parallel programs of instruction are carried out by the School of Nursing. Both undergraduate and graduate nursing students are trained in the basic medical and nursing techniques of the department. In addition, active on-the-job training for nursing personnel working in the department (registered nurses, practical nurses, and nursing assistants) has been organized by the department's nursing care coordinator.

For the past several summers, the hospital chaplain and the emergency department faculty have guided divinity school students in a course of counseling work for the families of patients in the department.

Both students and families have found this program beneficial in helping relatives cope with acute illness, trauma, or death.

HEALTH-CARE RESEARCH

The importance of research in the methods of health-care delivery has increased steadily as the health manpower crisis grows. The emergency department offers a testing ground that is well suited for this type of study. The faculty here is in a good position to initiate and to foster projects in this field.

At Strong Memorial Hospital a number of health-care studies have been undertaken. The most obvious of these involves an investigation of the problems requiring an emergency department facility. Our evaluation of the Strong Memorial Hospital emergency department indicates that 30% of the patients suffer from acute or life-threatening problems, that another 60% need attention within 24 hours and must use the department since no clinic or office visit could be arranged with such dispatch, and that about 10% could have received scheduled appointments at the convenience of the hospital. In evaluating this situation, we are agreed that a patient who feels an urgent need for care should see a physician, albeit briefly, whether or not the situation seems urgent to the doctor. A new Strong Memorial Hospital is currently under construction. We are reviewing these statistics concerning the public's use of the facility to plan the new emergency department.

A second project involves the work of psychiatric nurse clinicians. Two nurses who have received advanced nursing training in psychiatry coordinate the nursing care for psychiatric patients in the department. They guide the other nurses who are less skilled in psychiatric problems in the management of the acutely disturbed and possibly destructive patient. Working with the psychiatric resident in the department, they help with patient disposition, and they conduct some of the interview therapy in the department and in the follow-up clinic. They are supported by a social worker who also functions in the management of psychiatric emergencies. In this way the shortage of trained psychiatric personnel is at least partially alleviated.

Encouraged by the success of the psychiatric nurse clinician, the department is actively involved in the training of medical nurse practitioners. Some of the long delays in treating patients with nonurgent problems will be improved by utilizing a nurse practitioner to carry out initial evaluations and to render care under close supervision by a physician.

Two developments are being studied in the field of acute coronary care.

Mobile coronary care units. MCCUs are currently being established in this community. There is two-way radio communication between the emergency department and the ambulance, and the feasibility of transmitting electrocardiographic tracings to the emergency department has been demonstrated. Ambulance personnel are receiving intensive instruction in coronary care including techniques of heart-lung resuscitation, the nature of cardiac drugs, how to take an ECG, how to start I-V therapy and give I–V medication, and how to use a portable defibrillator. The Strong Memorial Hospital emergency department will be the communications center for the MCCU, and physicians there will monitor coronary patients being transported to any of the community hospitals. When the rhythm being monitored indicates that medication or defibrillation should be started, the ambulance attendants will be able to institute appropriate therapy on the doctor's order. Through an interhospital radio network, the emergency department can also communicate with the hospital emergency department to which the patient is being taken. The ECGs and the tape recordings of the communication between ambulance and the Strong Memorial Hospital physician will then be available to the receiving hospital. We are now in a position to study the impact of MCCUs on this community, and this should be done before a more extensive network of vehicles is obtained and more personnel trained.

Precoronary care units. Because of the large number of persons with chest pain who present to the emergency department each day, an area in the department has been established as a precoronary care unit. Here the patient with chest pain is initially evaluated. Proper monitoring equipment is available so that a definitive diagnosis can be made. If the chest pain is not due to a myocardial infarction, the patient can be discharged or admitted to an appropriate hospital floor. If, however, a myocardial infarction is diagnosed, the patient's therapy can be undertaken and his condition stabilized before he is transferred to the coronary intensive care unit. This study has demonstrated the importance of monitoring and defibrillating equipment with appropriately trained personnel in the emergency department.

Under the direction of the professor of medical education at the medical school, an investigation involving the use of television tapes as a teaching device was carried out. During the active management of an emergency patient, the episode was filmed. After proper editing, the tape was played back so that critical, constructive criticism of the management was possible. Interesting possibilities became evident for the use of this technique as a teaching device for medical students and house officers working in the department. The opportunity to review objectively what has been done during an emergency is much more vivid and intense when a pictorial record is available. This project has been shelved temporarily because of limited personnel and funds to maintain it. The potential for ongoing educational benefit is such, however, that we expect to resume the study at a later date.

SUMMARY

The emergency department is an important resource for education and health-care research in the medical center. If critical care of the acutely ill is to improve, a concerted effort must be made to improve teaching in this area. The emergency department is a dynamic institution. The community and hospital are constantly making new demands upon it. By the nature of emergency work, a staff and faculty flexible enough to accommodate these needs and demands are required. The faculty should be available to monitor the changing emergency scene, to recommend improvements, and to keep the teaching of emergency care current. Such teaching, then, is relevant and intellectually stimulating both to the students and to the faculty.

REFERENCES

[1] Goldfinger SE, Federman DD: Postgraduate education of community physicians, emergency care training in the emergency ward. JAMA 206:2883–2884, 1968

[2] Lucas CE, Ledgerwood A, Walt AJ: A scientific basis for medical student education in trauma. J Trauma 13:520–528, 1973

[3] Monaghan ED, Johnson G, Jr.: Guidelines for the education of medical students in emergency medical services. J Med Educ 48:1124–1128, 1973

[4] Morton JH and Lucria MN: An emergency department teaching program. J Med Educ 43:60–63, 1968

Robert H. Dailey

11

The Emergency Physician and His Residency Training

There is a trend in America toward the full-time practice of medicine within the hospital emergency department. The unusual demands of such practice have developed a unique consciousness and role for the emergency physician. The need for appropriately tailored training has been recognized and is now being answered by the rapid growth of residency programs. The problems and possibilities of such programs are examined in this chapter.

A METAPHOR

A new flower is growing in medicine's garden of specialties. Botanists argue whether it is a true flower or simply a weed. And even those claiming it [to be] a flower question its legitimacy, wondering whether it's simply a hybrid, formed by cross-pollination of other flowers in the garden. However, many classify it a genuinely new strain, its seed blown into the garden by the winds of necessity.

How has the flower been able to implant itself successfully in a garden already dense with other varieties? Astute observers have noted the flower takes root only in the most arid soils where other plants cannot and have not grown. Some fear it will crowd out and supplant the other flowers; but rather than displace, it appears to complement them, to fill gaps in the garden previously not even recognized.

Presently, there is a great controversy among ecologists: Some say the balance is being destroyed, that the new flower must be extirpated, while others suggest it should be nurtured as a beautiful and vigorous strain that lends both beauty and balance to the garden. The controversy continues, but the flower continues to grow and spread. So that now it remains to be seen only whether it will remain neglected as a runty sport, or whether instead, it will be cultivated, to blossom and become an accepted part of medicine's garden.

The flower in this metaphor is, of course, the emergency physician. The purpose of this chapter is to review his genesis, define his role, and examine the problems and possibilities of residency training programs.

Who is an emergency physician? The latest definition from "Standards for Residency Training Programs in Emergency Medicine" approved by the AMA House of Delegates is

> The emergency physician is one who is trained to engage in (1) the immediate initial recognition, evaluation, care, and disposition of patients in response to acute illness and injury; (2) the administration, research, and teaching of all aspects of emergency medical care; (3) the direction of the patient to sources of follow-up care, in or out of the hospital as may be required; (4) the provision when requested of emergency, but not continuing, care to in-hospital patients; and (5) the management of emergency medical systems for the provision of prehospital emergency care.

In a less conceptual and more realistic sense, we might better define him simply as "the doctor in the emergency department." Within this inelegant definition lies a very central point: whereas traditional specialists have defined themselves by patient age, sex, or pathologic condition, the emergency physician has rather been defined by patient needs in a changing pattern of delivery of primary medical care. Formerly, emergency departments were used relatively infrequently, and then most often for major sudden illnesses or injuries; they were manned by the entire hospital staff under duress on infrequent rotation. But now a new pattern is emerging: emergency departments are being used by large numbers of patients; these patients frequently have episodic problems of relatively minor nature; and they are attended by full-time emergency department physicians.

GENESIS OF THE EMERGENCY PHYSICIAN

Let us examine the factors operative upon the patient, the doctor, and the hospital that have promoted these changes.

Access to a family physician or other primary-care physician has become increasingly difficult for patients in the past 20 years. There are proportionately fewer general physicians, and the "family physician" is likely to be a specialist incapable of handling the wide spectrum of acute or episodic problems. Physicians are not available 24 hours a day, and they arrange night coverage by colleagues. Our modern society is increasingly mobile, so that people are becoming accustomed to, and often satisfied with, changing doctors and fragmented medical care. When there is no private physician immediately available, the emergency department becomes the logical alternative for episodic care. Finally, the increased sophistication of modern medicine has led to a decrease in house calls in favor of hospital-based care, where x-ray and laboratory services can be obtained and more definitive care rendered.

For the physician, full-time emergency medicine offers a career that is professionally stimulating and that provides a gratifying life-style. The doctor finds varied and challenging medical problems of a nonchronic nature. There is satisfactory remuneration. Since the hospital provides his office, ancillary personnel, and professional supplies, overhead is relatively low. He has frequent contact with the whole spectrum of in-depth specialists whom he can consult and thus obtain ongoing professional education. This practice assures regular hours and undisturbed free time; the physician may plan vacations with ease and free conscience.

There are definite advantages for hospitals to have emergency departments and also to staff them with full-time emergency physicians. First, the myth of unprofitable emergency departments has been exploded. The emergency department is an excellent means for hospitals to compete for inpatients; these inpatients in turn tend to be sicker, and hospitalization is more lengthy than elective admissions; their presence in special care units generates a disproportionately large amount of inpatient revenues. The numbers of patients seeking emergency care have skyrocketed in the past decades, making the emergency department more efficient. Also, increasing numbers of people are being covered by private, state, or federal third-party insurance, insurance that almost always covers emergency visits; this reduces bad debt. Increasing medical sophistication has led to a real disparity between theoretically possible care and available care, thus raising the specter of malpractice; therefore, hospitals are increasingly turning to full-time emergency physicians who assure the commitment, competence, and administrative continuity that decrease chances of medicolegal actions.

Most of these pressures will probably continue in the future, cementing an increasing demand for emergency physicians. Concomitantly, emergency physicians are increasing in numbers and influence. They have formed national organizations, such as the American College of Emergency Physicians, and the University Association for Emergency Medical Services, which are close to achieving specialty status, and are now pressing for formal education in this field. Medical schools are responding by increasing curriculum time in Emergency Medicine for medical students and also by initiating Emergency Medicine residency programs: more than 30 are now operative.

These pressures and trends seem to assure a place in medicine for the Emergency Physician. If this is the case, what is his professional role in contrast to that of more traditional physicians?

ROLE OF THE EMERGENCY PHYSICIAN

Although it is not our purpose to defend emergency medicine as a specialty, special education for the emergency physician presupposes a unique role in medical practice. Let us examine his patients, his decision making, the milieu of the emergency department, and the goals of patient care.

The Emergency Department is a special workshop, very different from an office or hospital ward. The patients are unscheduled and alternately too few and too many; some of them are upset, unruly, obtunded, in pain, or otherwise unable to cooperate or give a coherent history; some need immediate attention, and others demand it; most are previously unknown to the doctor and are being seen at one brief time in the natural history of disease. The old records or prior medical history are often unavailable; evaluation is performed in an area frequently cramped, crowded, chaotic, and noisy; the physician is often hurried and harried; there may be only limited laboratory and x-ray support; and consultative services may be hours away.

To function in this milieu requires a special approach by the emergency physician. He must quickly establish rapport, focus on the patient's major problem, aggressively seek ancillary information sources, be aware of the patient's immediate home and social situation, have a keen understanding of natural history of disease, be able to perform rapid pertinent physical examination, and not depend heavily on sophisticated laboratory and x-ray services. Minor obvious problems can be diagnosed and treated, but with more critically ill patients he must concentrate on a logical understanding of the phenomenon presented and correct its pathophysiology. Thus, in critical patients the watchwords are *define* and *stabilize*, rather than necessarily diagnose and treat. Most important is the ability to decide "sick or not sick"; "keep or discharge." Finally, to effect appropriate disposition, the emergency physician must know the total medical and social resources of the hospital and community.

As well as working in a different environment that demands a different approach, the actual clinical and nonclinical content of his knowledge and skills is also in many ways unique. Let us examine this content in the context of our original metaphorical emergency physician depicted as a flower in Figure 11.1.

The parts of this flower are depicted semiquantitatively. The roles

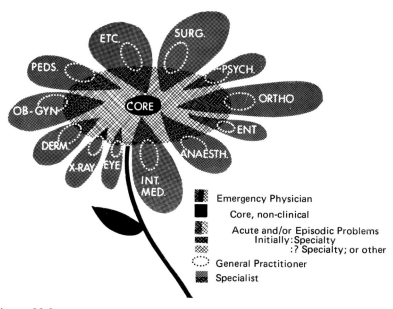

Figure 11.1
Emergency physician depicted as a flower.

of the emergency physician, general practitioner, and in-depth specialist are contrasted. The flower encompasses all three areas, the emergency physician being represented by the large cross-hatched oval area. Acute and episodic care falls within this oval; chronic and long-term care outside of it. Each in-depth specialist is represented by a petal of the flower, the general practitioner by the sum total of smaller enclosed areas within the petals. Note that most of the concerns of the general practitioner and specialist are chronic and long-term and only a small part, acute and episodic.

The emergency physician's domain is divided basically into clinical and nonclinical areas, the large outer and small inner ovals, respectively. Let us deal with the clinical area first. Some acute problems are easy to classify in a given specialty area; for example, the asthmatic (internal medicine). A considerable portion of patient presentations in emergency departments are phenomena, however, and not initially specialty diagnoses. These patients need evaluation before being specialty-relegated; for example, patients with hematuria which could be either medical or urologic. Some patients have more than one acute problem, thus involving more than one specialist; for example, the multiple injury patient sustaining fractured extremities, blunt abdominal trauma, and head injury (the "trauma team" patient). Some problems simply do not fall easily into any specialty category and are seen almost exclusively in the emergency department: Rape, toothache, weekend venereal disease, fishhooks, dog bite, exposure, drowning, overdoses, industrial and recreational injuries, and acute psychosis or situational reactions are only a few examples. Finally, in a strictly practical vein, there are those "specialty" problems for which there is no immediately available specialist. Thus, since the emergency physician must handle it, ventricular tachycardia with shock legitimately becomes his province in the absence of a cardiologist. Practically, there is no consultation for true emergencies.

The central oval, labeled *core*, represents nonclinical areas that are unique to the emergency physician. These represent a wide variety of administrative skills and knowledge of community out-reach services that must be mastered by the emergency physician for him to be effective in the emergency department. Consider the following specific examples: medicolegal implications of rape, crimes of violence, drug and alcohol abuse, and coroner cases; ambulance services; extrication and rescue; emergency communications; safety and accident prevention programs, hospital and area-wide disaster planning and execution; and city, county, and state laws regarding delivery of emergency services. Figure 11.2 represents the central role of the emergency department as "clearinghouse" for such problems and services.

148

City, County, State and Federal Administration

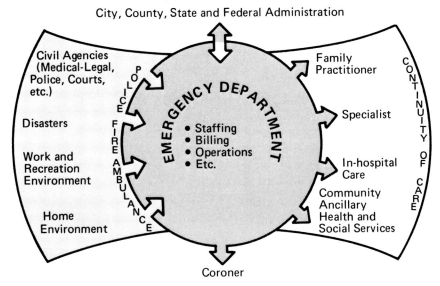

Figure 11.2
Emergency department as a clearinghouse.

Thus, the emergency physician should have a unique core of administrative knowledge, plus a body of clinical skills and knowledge that are applied by him in a manner unique to the emergency department.

TRAINING OF THE EMERGENCY PHYSICIAN: PROBLEMS AND CHALLENGES

At the present time, we are faced with hundreds of emergency departments in the United States staffed by physicians without adequate formal training to be entirely effective there. These physicians are of diverse professional backgrounds, and they must have available postgraduate education fitting their individual needs. Additionally, many medical students and house officers are planning to make emergency medicine a life-long career. In the remainder of this chapter proposals for necessary residency programs will be outlined. The what (curriculum), where (hospital locale), how (teaching method), and by whom (faculty) must be determined. Let us deal with each of these challenges separately.

Curriculum planning is a necessity, an opportunity, and a very difficult task. The American College of Emergency Physicians has made a start in attempting to define emergency medicine. Working from its definition of the emergency physician, this organization has devised

149

and revised "Essentials for Graduate Education (Residency) of Emergency Physicians." It recommends 3 years of training following graduation from medical school. The following requirements have recently been determined by the Graduate Education Committee of the College for approval of such residency programs. In the most general terms the clinical content should include emergency aspects of internal medicine (including CCU and medical ICU), surgery, orthopedics, pediatrics, plastic surgery, thoracic surgery, neurology and neurosurgery, obstetrics-gynecology, psychiatry, radiology, urology, opthalmology, ENT, anesthesia, and dentistry. Time for research, electives, and for the non-clinical areas, as previously described, should be allocated. During the training program, annual examination of the resident is required; residents less than 24 months in training after medical school must be directly supervised by a senior emergency resident or staff physician while working in the Emergency Department.

Within these broad guidelines, however, a detailed list of requisite knowledge and skills must be developed by consensus of those initiating and participating in emergency residency programs. The courses of study (curricula) that should evolve directly from such activity will have to vary greatly in response to local facilities, patient flow loads, departmental strengths and weaknesses, etc. All should teach basically the same things, however, if not necessarily in the same way! Further, in contrast to other specialties, a disproportionate amount of teaching must be directed to acute and crisis problems (*e.g.*, airway and circulatory support). Even though they represent a minority of patient representations, their occurrence is where expertise spells the difference between mortality and survival.

How then is such training to be achieved? A crucial problem has been academic medicine's traditional lack of participation in the Emergency Department. This can be explained by a real disparity in the aims and interests of traditional academic specialty departments and the emergency department. First, emergency department patients do not belong to any single specialty, and the patients must be "sorted and labeled" before specialty interests are engendered. Further, specialties are disease oriented, not problem oriented; they concentrate in-depth rather than in-breadth; they concentrate more on inpatients than outpatients; more on secondary care than primary care; and in universities they are oriented more toward research and basic science than toward patient service. Finally, quite simply, emergency aspects are rightfully only a part of their total care concerns. All these discrepancies, however, must be squared with the need for emergency medicine education.

A second great problem of emergency medicine education is the inferior administrative, physical, and staffing situation of the emergency department. It is seldom accorded hospital departmental status, existing instead as a section or division of some other department (or worse yet, simply as the "emergency service"). It is overseen either by a committee or by a junior member of some other department under duress. Lacking a champion, it cannot compete with other departments for the necessities of life, *i.e.*, space, monies, and staff. Accordingly, we find reluctant junior house staff delivering hasty care in cramped quarters without direct staff supervision. Clearly, such a setting is not appropriate for physician training.

Alternatively, should we then train an emergency physician on various specialty services? There are theoretic difficulties and there have been practical difficulties in this approach: The trainee is likely to get an experience that is largely inappropriate to his eventual practice situation; it is a brief exposure in a lengthy program designed for another specialist; he is a "second-class citizen" or "guest"; he must adapt himself to the needs of the service rather than vice versa; didactic teaching is necessarily directed to the needs of the specialty residents; there is no way to structure his training in a logical fashion, that is, critical skills first; once "off" a given service, vital knowledge and skills are forgotten as he joins a totally different service. Finally, in essence, he loses his sense of identity as an emergency physician.

One of the most uncomfortable questions faced in emergency medicine training is "Who will teach this new specialty?" No currently existing physician is completely adequate. The conscientious general physician who has practiced emergency medicine for some time has a great deal of practical expertise but less than ideal in-depth sophistication; the rare specialist who has extensive emergency department experience offers only narrow expertise; and the university-based academician, who can contribute greatly to understanding pathophysiology, has little or no practical emergency department experience.

This array of training problems both within and without the emergency department cannot be lightly considered or dismissed. But the problems themselves suggest solutions.

TRAINING OF THE EMERGENCY PHYSICIAN: PROPOSALS

The training of the emergency physician must begin in medical school. There should be a part of all 4 years devoted to training in emergency medicine. This training might include in the first year some orientation to community emergency medical services and instruction in first-aid. As the student progresses, he should be instructed in the basics of rapid patient evaluation, problem identification, and disposition services. Finally, he should become familiar with principles of care of acute illness and injury. Appropriate separate curriculum time should be set aside each year. Such might be done by departments separately or, preferably, in concert (an emergency care curriculum).

For both the medical student and the postgraduate physician, the emergency department should be made the most suitable place for training. A suitable place must have an adequate flow of acutely ill and injured patients and all the services and space for their adequate care. Full-time, academically inclined staff physicians must be recruited for teaching and supervision. These physicians might well be a mix of emergency physicians and in-depth specialists from other departments with emergency experience, thus providing both breadth and depth to the teaching program.

The emergency department should be made a separate administrative department, thus being able to vie on an even footing with other hospital departments for space, monies, and staff. In university hospitals, particularly those with large emergency departments, strong consideration should be given to the idea of separate academic departmental status. This status would provide the commitment, concentration of faculty, and emphasis for teaching all levels of emergency personnel. It is also highly desirable that other specialty residents participate in emergency department care. This participation is a valid experience for the resident in emergency care of the patient in his specialty; at a senior level he can act as a specialty consultant; and he can then better understand the possibilities and constraints of emergency medicine. Finally, a mutually educational relationship can exist between the emergency physician trainee and the specialty resident.

Even with a large, well-functioning emergency department, there will always have to be training in such units as the MICU, CCU, and certain appropriate specialty departments. Great flexibility should be exercised in the use of the emergency department and these other departments. It would also seem ideal that training be provided in a number of different institutions, that is, community hospitals, university hospitals, and county hospitals, since each provides experiences not obtainable in the others, but all of which are necessary.

Once a curriculum is developed for training, there should be instruction in the most critical skills and knowledge early in the program; thus in the first few months the following must be covered: Cardiopulmonary resuscitation, airway management, evaluation and treatment of shock states, major trauma priorities, control of hemorrhage, and treatment of medical emergencies, such as pulmonary edema and asthma. How should such subjects be taught? Most importantly, evaluating and caring for patients in the setting of real responsibility and with adequate free time for concurrent reading about these problems is probably the most crucial part of any residency experience. The emphasis must center on real patient-care responsibility and resident responsibility for self-education. Care must be taken to provide training in the previously listed nonclinical areas which involve the physician in the community. Knowledge of areas outside the hospital, such as the coroner's office, public health facilities, and fire and police departments are necessary. Seminars can be held by people involved in emergency department staffing, financing, and administration. Residents should become actively involved in such areas in order to deal in-depth with such particular aspects of EMS delivery.

Conference time, free of service obligations, must be set aside. This time can either be in slack hours (such as early morning) or when a double-staffing pattern is provided by overlap at shift time. These conferences should actively involve the trainee by prereading before lectures, by presenting cases or didactic materials, by performing simulations or procedures on manikins, cadaver, or animal material, etc. Case-related sessions are excellent, such as emergency department death reviews, morning chart reviews, and Clinical Pathologic Conferences. Acute care crises can be captured on videotape and later reviewed.

Follow-up of emergency patients is necessary to judge the adequacy of emergency department care and develop an understanding of the natural history of disease. This can be obtained by rounding on inpatients, contacting inpatient staff for follow-up, receiving discharge summaries of all admitted patients, retrieving charts of patients referred to outpatient clinics, and allowing follow-up emergency department visits for selected patients (*e.g.*, wound and cast checks).

Until there are a greater number of journals devoted to emergency medicine, some mechanism must be used to capture pertinent developments in the literature. To this end a large number of journals can regularly be scanned jointly by staff and residents and useful articles reported in a journal club format. These articles, plus appropriate audiovisual aids, books, photographic slides, and x-ray films should form the basis of a department library.

Cooperation between emergency physician residency programs all over the nation must be encouraged to share the inevitable growth pains. It is hoped that teaching materials, residents, and ideas may be exchanged. Man-hours in development will remain particularly precious during our development phase.

Recently, ACEP and UA/EMS jointly have formed the Liaison Residency Endorsement Committee to assist emerging residencies in promoting quality education. This committee's endorsement procedure will be supplanted by traditional AMA review if and when emergency medicine becomes an AMA-recognized specialty.

Although the thrust of this article deals primarily with resident training, for many years in the future we must provide suitable educational experience for physicians from other specialties who desire to change in mid-course to emergency medicine. Therefore, a variety of postgraduate experiences must be designed that go far beyond the present postgraduate lecture courses. The problem-oriented approach, games, simulations, videotapes, etc., should all be considered. Self-assessment testing can be used to tailor intensive emergency medicine training. Those physicians with surgical backgrounds should be given medical training, physicians with medical backgrounds should be given surgical training. Clinical courses for 1, 2, and 3 weeks can be designed to give physicians critical bedside skills and knowledge. One-half year or yearly fellowships could be offered.

If these undertakings seem ambitious, it must not be forgotten that other emergency health-care professionals must be trained: nurses, ambulance attendants, paramedics, physician's assistants, etc. All of these people can considerably substitute for and extend the services of the emergency physician.

A great deal of plain hard work lies ahead in emergency medicine. If it is mixed with like amounts of flexibility, originality, and real patient orientation in the design of emergency residency programs, we shall greatly upgrade primary acute care in the United States.

Paul A. Ebert

12

Training of the Emergency Physician

The discussion of training of residents from medicine or surgery in the emergency department must be considered under the broadest guidelines. At a time when emergency departments are undergoing considerable revamping and developing programs to train physicians especially for work in the emergency departments, the roles of traditional departments of medicine and surgery become less clearly defined. The reader commonly relates any attempt to define educational programs with his own local situation and thus may note considerable variations with the educational views expressed. Without question, specialty departments such as medicine and surgery must maintain adequate input to insure that their residents are reasonably experienced in the problems of the emergency department.

In discussing the operational features of emergency rooms, it would seem that today three basic structures commonly exist in the teaching hospital.

First, the emergency department is operated by one of the traditional specialties of the hospital, most commonly surgery, and has undergone little change in the past decade.

Second, the emergency department is still operated by one of the traditional specialties, such as medicine, surgery, or possibly family practice, but full-time physicians are being integrated and may provide the majority of primary care in the department.

Third, the emergency department is operated by an emergency department physician, and an additional group of physicians is under him. In this situation, traditional specialists, such as those in medicine and surgery, are consultants to the emergency department and may participate at the advisory committee level for the operation of the department, but they may provide little, if any, primary care.

Emergency departments have adopted various administrative structures, and the wide variety exists primarily because of the different demands made on emergency facilities. For example, one hospital may operate a very active trauma service and thus have the need for considerable surgical input at the primary care level. In another, the number of trauma cases may be minimal, whereas the number of walk-in, nonacute problems may be exhaustive. In the one setting, a group of physicians well versed in the management of emergencies, principles of resuscitation, blood replacement, and rapid movement to the surgical theater is paramount for good patient management. In the other setting, the emergency department may closely parallel an ambulatory care facility that handles a large number of nonurgent walk-in patients. Obviously, the educational requirements of each of these groups are entirely different, and the training available to a resident in either setting also varies from one extreme to another. It is easy to understand how a department of surgery would operate an emergency department having a large volume of trauma, whereas a department handling primarily nonurgent ambulatory patients could be organized very poorly by the department of surgery.

It seems impossible, and probably undesirable, to standardize emergency departments, since the department must respond to the needs of the community and to the type of population it serves. Thus the structure of residency training will vary considerably from hospital to hospital, and the input and availability of teaching experience for residents in medicine and surgery are going to vary considerably. Yet as we move more toward staffing by emergency department physicians, we must demand that specialty training in medicine, surgery, pediatrics, etc., have adequate exposure to the emergency situation. It would be entirely wrong to eliminate emergency experience from the traditional specialty residency programs. It would not be long before a generation of pediatricians, internists, or surgeons existed who would not be adequately trained in any form of acute care.

TRAINING TRADITIONAL SPECIALISTS
IN THE EMERGENCY DEPARTMENT

It seems easier to discuss postgraduate medical or surgical training in hospitals that do not have emergency department physicians since the entire primary care could be performed by these specialists. This structure poses no particular problems in administration or education; therefore, it can be discussed under the routine format of residency training in which an associated training program for the emergency department physician exists. It would seem important that all primary care not be designated exclusively to the emergency physician training program when the emergency facility is staffed entirely by emergency department physicians. Some positions should be available for specialists in medicine, pediatrics, surgery, and other specialties to obtain experience in primary emergency department care. Thus close interaction between the departments will be necessary, and, even though a current pressing demand for emergency department physicians is apparent, it is probably imprudent to attempt to solve this manpower demand by total exclusion of other specialties from emergency care. There must be some sharing of the educational resources, and in a properly supervised emergency department residency program, a rotation of other specialists through this facility under the direction of the emergency department would be most meaningful. Obviously, the total amount of clinical material available will be a major factor, and in most medical or surgical programs this will result in less experience per resident.

ORGANIZATION

It is not the purpose of this chapter to address itself to the organizational structure of the emergency department. Some mention should be made, however, since it has direct bearing on the educational programs that will be available within the department. One of the major problems in the past has been the large service needs of many emergency departments and the solving of these service demands by so-called residency training experience. In some emergency departments where the majority of care is provided by residents on a month-to-month basis, it has not been possible to establish guidelines or goals or to alter significantly the patterns of delivering emergency services. Delay in seeing patients, diagnosis errors, and patients' dissatisfaction with the service have been common complaints. All emergency departments involved in any form of residency training should have a defined full-time director. Depending upon the size of the facility and the volume of patients seen, additional full-time members of the department are desirable. An advisory committee to the director should be composed of traditional specialties, so that input into care, education, programs, and direction of the department is available.

RESIDENCY TRAINING

The following comments regarding residency training in the emergency department will be directed primarily toward the departments of medicine and surgery, although many of the philosophic aspects are applicable to other departments. This outline is not directed toward the training of the emergency department physician. The traditional educational experience of a resident in the emergency department from medicine or surgery has been subjected to many criticisms. The amount of time spent in the emergency department has been short since this training represents only a fraction of the entire residency training. Depending upon the emergency room environment, it may provide a very limited experience in true emergency care. For this reason it is most important that some form of structured didactic program exist to be certain of adequate coverage of the subject material. In many instances the specialty resident is not particularly interested in emergency care because he does not see this as occupying a major portion of his career goal. Yet the exposure to acutely ill patients is a common, everyday experience in both hospital and office practice. The type of patients seen in an emergency facility is often repetitious and nonurgent, and these patients are often unwilling to undergo specific diagnostic studies during the operation of the usual ambulatory care facility. Thus the resident is faced with a high percentage of patients for whom he feels adequate services are available through other ambulatory facilities of the hospital, and the patient should not be seen in the emergency department. This common situation does not necessarily negate good patient care or good educational experience for the trainee.

TRAINING PROGRAM

At what stage in training should the resident rotate through the emergency department to obtain the best educational experience? There usually are two opinions on this question, and both answers have merit.

Early Training

The resident should be exposed to emergency care very early in his training because it is an opportunity to participate actively in patient care and to make a large number of independent decisions. The number of experiences is so large in a concentrated period of time that it gives the individual an opportunity to mature at an earlier phase of training.

Later Training

The opposite approach is that the person should go to the emergency department after 1 or 2 years of training because the resident is asked to make many independent and rapid decisions; he has fewer laboratory and diagnostic tests to use before arriving at an initial decision; the number of patients seen in the department is so large that a more experienced physician can handle the number more effectively; and the responsibility is greater, so the emergencies are handled better by a more experienced resident. Personally, the author favors the second approach because the emergency department is such an important aspect of our total health-care system, and more efficient management is required. We do need to insure the best quality of care and let education be an outgrowth of it.

When an emergency department residency program exists, the rotation of a second- or third-year medical or surgical resident offers additional expertise in the respective specialized areas. Therefore, more mutual interchange between residents and staff should benefit both programs. This system would seem to support and improve an emergency physician program and yet allow adequate experience in primary emergency care to the rotating specialist. It is apparent that, in programs with a training program for emergency department physicians, the experience of the traditional specialty residents will be lessened. Thus the need for a "core" didactic program is more important since the direct patient educational experience per resident is likely to decrease.

STRUCTURED PROGRAM

Either as a continual program during the entire year or as a structured program during the emergency department experience, certain specific areas need be presented in a didactic and probably repetitious format. Certain categoric areas, such as medical, pediatric, gynecologic, and surgical emergencies, should be presented by each specialty. General principles in the management of shock, fluid replacement, hemodynamics, cardiac resuscitation, tracheal intubation, etc., need to be emphasized.

Input by the emergency service of the local fire or police departments, routine first-aid without specialized equipment, and psychological aspects of trauma and injury need be presented in a didactic program. Obviously, these lectures, discussions, or seminars have little meaning without adequate clinical experience or teaching. A properly prepared resident will be more efficient, learn more from the clinical experience, and have considerably more confidence in his judgment if the above general topics have been well covered prior to the resident's experience in the emergency department.

To increase the experience per resident, it is suggested that daily service chart rounds be held each day at the changing of staff. The majority of patients are routine, but several patients with management problems are usually seen every day in even the less busy emergency department. These sessions allow considerable discussion among residents from different services and exchange of views on similar problems.

The structuring of time so that all residents can rotate simultaneously through, or have available, an outpatient facility allows a return visit by a patient to the same physician who saw him in the emergency department. There is no better way to learn from a decision made in the urgent situation than to see the patient in return visit to evaluate the effects of the initial treatment and accuracy of diagnosis.

LENGTH OF ROTATION

There is no ideal amount of time a resident needs to rotate through an emergency service to gain a useful experience. In general a majority of programs have had a rotation of 2–3 months in an emergency department. If the department is reasonably busy, this certainly should be adequate exposure to gain competence in urgent care. There are several considerations for the future that may affect the experience of the specialty resident rotating through the emergency department. With more full-time emergency department physicians providing a considerable portion of primary care, there will be less need for resident services in the emergency room and, thus, fewer educational opportunities for the resident in this environment. Therefore, we are beginning a period of change in the pattern of emergency care education, and the optimal solution is not known at this time.

Specialist and Resident Experience

It is apparent that a resident's educational experience will undoubtedly intertwine closely with a full-time emergency department specialist, and the amount of independent experience per resident will undoubtedly be limited. One might argue that with more and more emergency departments having full-time coverage, it is not necessary to teach emergency care to medical and surgical residents. This idea seems unrealistic since most specialists need to be involved in organizing and planning the treatment of any patient suffering an emergent situation from the time the patient arrives at the hospital. This continuation of education in patient care is needed to allow a medical or surgical resident to understand the problem the initial physician faces in dealing with many truly emergent conditions. This continuation does not mean that he is going to deliver this primary emergent care in most emergency departments in the future, but his participation in improving and setting standards for high-quality emergent care is needed. The next few years appear to provide an interesting aspect in emergency department education in regard to an emergency department specialist and the traditional surgical and medical residents who also must gain educational experience in this environment. Each institution will undoubtedly evolve some type of working arrangement, but every effort must be made to insure that the length of time a traditional specialty resident rotates in the emergency department is sufficient to gain reasonable competence in understanding acute illness.

Ongoing Training

One of the greatest deficiencies in most of our residency systems is the lack of continued emphasis on education after the initial rotation through the emergency department. A difficulty in our residency training programs is that emergency medicine or surgery is to be learned in the emergency department rotation and that no structured continual educational experience is available to the resident through the entire period of training. Educational programs in acute care should be ongoing throughout the year for each year of the resident's training. As mentioned, it is impossible to cover each emergent situation in a short rotation through a service, and a great number of these situations need to be reemphasized during each year of a maturing educational experience.

EMERGENCY SERVICES TO THE COMMUNITY

One of our greatest gaps between the physician and the active community is the relationship between the emergency services of the community and the hospital. In many cities a very excellent emergency service is available through either the fire or the police departments, and many well-trained paramedics are employed by these services. Involving these community emergency services in a periodic demonstration program with the graduate training program is of paramount importance.

The doctor must be aware of the types of service available to patients and the potential capabilities of these services. Thus, several demonstrations per year to the specialty residents are of great importance in their education, and input from the residents through the emergency service can be of value. It is probably not practical to rotate residents on an ambulance service in most of the major cities. A very short rotation such as this would have immense educational value for the resident but has little practical importance to the future delivery of health service. When time and circumstances permit, this rotation undoubtedly is an invaluable experience to a specialty resident.

It is apparent that trying to describe the residency training in the emergency department is not possible on a broad scale. It is obvious that considerable change in the educational opportunities for medical and surgical residents is forthcoming. With the development of residency programs for emergency department physicians and more full-time emergency-room personnel, there will obviously be a decrease in educational opportunity for the traditional specialty residents. Thus it is important that forms of didactic teaching be structured through the entire specialty residency. A well-prepared resident is apt to gain considerably more experience from a limited rotation than one that has not been prepared prior to the rotation through the emergency department. Therefore, program directors must consider developing other types of teaching mechanisms for which clinical situations could be simulated and the resident required to make an evaluation and provide a practical approach to the presented problem. As medical care becomes more regionalized with emergency trauma services localized to certain hospitals, other forms of educational experiences, whether they are rotations through busy services or simulated clinical settings, will have to be developed to provide a broad experience in emergency medicine.

W. F. Bouzarth

13

Training the "Second-Career" Emergency Physician

Many factors have continued to focus greater attention on the otherwise neglected area of emergency medical services: first, the disappearance of the general practitioner; second, the vanishing internship; and third, the advent of the emergency room as a major point at which the public now enters the health delivery care system. More physicians are needed to man the "pit." To make the position attractive, the emergency physician is offered more money than was given his predecessors, less time on duty, paid vacations, and other fringe benefits. Establishment of the American College of Emergency Physicians, a trend to develop the emergency room into a department, and the development of residency programs in emergency medicine now offer status to this position. It is a small wonder that those physicians weary of the trials and tribulations of private practice seek shelter in the emergency area. The qualifications of these physicians who choose a "second career" in emergency medicine may come in question. Is a surgeon who has developed Parkinsonism and cannot operate qualified to treat a patient with acute pulmonary edema caused by a myocardial infarction? Can a cardiologist who is unable to hear a third heart sound because of otosclerosis perform peritoneal lavage in a patient with blunt abdominal trauma? Will the anesthesiologist who is retired because of hemorrhoids offer proper emergency care for an open fracture of the femur? Finally, does the once-too-busy general practitioner who has "retired" to the emergency room insert an endotracheal tube in an unconscious head-injured patient with speed and dispatch? With few exceptions, the answer to these questions is a resounding no.

Another problem rears its ugly head: Will second-career physicians, who are usually a proud group, admit their deficiencies and correct them? To judge by the overflow attendance at medical meetings devoted to emergency subjects, the answer is yes. Didactic presentations, however, do not develop manipulative skills. Except for an additional internship, fellowship, or residency, what recourse does the emergency physician have to train himself better? Of course, he can learn endotracheal intubation in the anesthesia department in his own hospital, but this apparently has certain drawbacks. What appears to be needed— perhaps on a national scale—is the development of a short course on emergency problems giving didactic and practical clinical experience. The Harvard 2-week course does just that, but it does not stress trauma.[3]

COURSES IN EMERGENCY MEDICINE

In 1970 the Pennsylvania Medical Society concerned itself with this problem.[1] Three workshops were held with representatives from six Pennsylvania medical schools and other groups as noted in Table 13.1. It was concluded that 2–3 week courses cannot be expected to be definitive. They can, however, build on prior knowledge, strengthen manipulative skills, and point out areas of deficiency. From there, the emergency physician can meet specific needs with further continuing educational programs.

To fulfill this obligation, quickly graded tests must be devised, perhaps integrated with a computer,[4] to inform the physician of his deficiencies at the beginning of the course. More importantly, with the use of a repeat test at the end of the course, the physician can be told how much he has improved and in what areas he still needs work.

Table 13.1. Organizations Represented at Workshops

Medical schools	Other organizations
Hahnemann Medical College	American College of Emergency Physicians
Harvard University	
	American College of Surgeons
Milton S. Hershey Medical Center	Greater Delaware Valley Regional Medical Program
Medical College of Pennsylvania	Pennsylvania Department of Health
Temple University	
	Susquehanna Valley Regional Medical Program
Thomas Jefferson University	
University of Cincinnati	U.S. Public Health Service
University of Pennsylvania	
University of Pittsburgh	

Three-Week Courses

Analysis of the various Pennsylvania workshops indicates that 3 weeks is the minimum time required to begin the retraining of an emergency physician. The 3 weeks should be arranged either en bloc or over a 3-year period, 1 week at a time, the former being preferable. This course should cost about $200 a week, fulfill the requirements for the American Medical Association's recognition award, and include a written appraisal by the faculty. To be successful, such programs require close cooperation between medical schools and large teaching hospitals.

Didactic and Practical Training

After a great deal of discussion, it was agreed that 25% of the week's instruction should be didactic and 75% should be devoted to practical experience in the emergency department, anesthesia and surgical suite, delivery room, intensive care unit, and cardiac care unit. In every area, especially the emergency department, the physician-student should be assigned to a specific preceptor(s). These preceptors must be paid. There is some advantage to assigning each physician-student to the same preceptor.

Practical instruction in these areas would not be prearranged, but would be governed, to a certain extent, by the type of problems presented by incoming patients and by the need of the physician-student. Each week's program would cover approximately 60 hours. Development of independent judgment by the trainee would be the major objective in the emergency department experience.

Patient flow. From the three courses given in Pennsylvania to date, it appears that the physician-student should be trained in an emergency department with a minimum volume of 50,000 visits per year. Even with that, there will be lulls in patient flow. An audit should be conducted to determine the frequency of visits during the week so that the trainee can budget his time to be in the emergency department at the height of its activity. This peak is usually in the evening; consequently, the traditional pattern of daytime instruction may need to be abandoned.

Study materials. To help fill the unavoidable slowdowns in emergency department activity, study materials should be provided. These materials may include a teaching manual, video cassettes, slide-sound sets, and computer interactions. Required reading of textbooks or reprints probably takes away from this program, although the physician-student should have this resource for reference. It is important that the preceptor be available during lull periods to answer questions and go over the administrative problems. It is also advisable to organize the hospital's regular continuing education programs during the 3-week course to emphasize emergency-type subjects. For example, if a diabetic specialist is to talk on the treatment of insulin coma, he should be scheduled during this 3-week period in preference, perhaps, to a lecturer on muscular dystrophy.

Emergency manipulative skills. Manipulative skills for emergency physicians have been outlined.[2] It is unrealistic to assume such an exhaustive list could be mastered in a short time. Therefore, the Pennsylvania course concentrated upon the first hour of emergency care. For example, relieving a tension pneumothorax was considered more important than teaching the physician-student sigmoidoscopy; however, the trainee would more likely be observing and performing the latter during the course. It is for this reason that an active emergency department is a prerequisite for any second-career course since it is impossible to schedule emergencies. Nevertheless, by cooperating with active in-service departments, the physician-student can learn to perform certain emergency skills that are otherwise routine. For example, one physician-student was assigned to the neurosurgical service to learn to pass a central venous catheter (a "routine" procedure for all intracranial operations), the art of inserting a needle into the lumbar subarachnoid space (he also learned the contraindications of lumbar puncture), and the importance of the mini-neurologic examination.

Life-Support Week

To concentrate on a certain aspect of emergency medicine, the 3-week course was divided into life support, trauma, and medical emergencies. The life-support week stressed noninvasive airway support. The operating suite offered an excellent opportunity for the physician-student to learn endotracheal intubation. In fact, to master this particular manipulative skill time was set aside in the second and third weeks as the trainee required. The life-support week included cardiac arrhythmias and ECG interpretation. The physician-student was encouraged to observe the cardiac resuscitation team in action and to participate if cardiac arrest occurred in the emergency department. This participation, too, was considered an integral part of the trauma and medical training. Table 13.2 lists the didactic curricula.

Trauma Week

The trauma week stressed surgical emergencies including subspecialty care. It was not difficult to take advantage of routine procedures for emergency-type training. One physician-student felt inadequate in suturing a laceration and was not desirous of learning "in front of" patients. The surgical resident arranged for him to scrub in at the end of operative procedures to help close surgical wounds. Soon the physician-student could tie a square knot, but more importantly, he could now concentrate on the most neglected part of traumatic wound care— proper debridement. During this week the trainees might also perform pelvic examination in the operating room prior to routine gynecologic procedures, and might relearn proper delivery techniques on the obstetric floor.

Medical-Emergency Week

The third week stressed medical and other special emergencies. One physician-student had little exposure to pediatric problems. Arrangements were made for much of his time to be spent at a pediatric

Table 13.2. Outline of Didactic Curricula

Life support	Surgical	Medical
Steps on the pathway from life to death	Wound care and prophylaxis	Acute myocardial infarctions and associated arrythmias
Airway control	ENT and dental problems	Alcoholism, drug abuse, and poisons
Practice session/airway control equipment	Thoracic injuries	Gastrointestinal bleeding
Physiology of respiratory systems	Neurosurgical emergencies	Pneumonia, venereal disease, infections, and antibiotics (2 hours)
Signs and symptoms management	Acute problems of the abdomen	Acute phychosis
Practice session	Fractures and dislocations (vascular insufficiency)	Nontraumatic shock
Cardiac arrest (emergency treatment, prolonged treatment)	Eye injuries	Neurologic emergencies and convulsions
Circulatory collapse and shock	Abdominal injuries	Pediatric emergencies (problems of the newborn)
Cardiac rhythm disturbances	Obstetric-gynecologic emergencies	Thromboembolism and hemorrhagic problems
Areawide EMS organization	Wounds of the face and hand	Congestive heart failure and pulmonary edema
Problems of rescue and extrication	Burns and vascular injuries	Metabolic emergencies
Proper ambulance design and equipment	Traumatic shock (etiology, diagnosis, control of bleeding, how to treat)	Asthma, allergy, and anaphylaxis
Emergency medical technician	Indications and contraindications for x-ray procedures	Hypertensive crisis
Triage	Priorities in the injured	Roundtable discussion/wrap-up
Practice session/problem of extrication, etc.	Roundtable discussion/wrap-up	

hospital. Drug abuse and alcoholism, two prevalent epidemic diseases, are stressed during this week. Interpretation of x-ray films, the emergency treatment of hypertensive crisis, and the differential diagnosis of coma were taught in the didactic sessions.

Administrative Procedures

By the end of the course the physician-students were more capable of managing emergencies, but what about administrative problems? It had been suggested that this be a subject of a fourth week. Instead the workshop participants concluded that a few hours should be devoted each week to this important subject, and practical experience could be obtained by observing administrative procedures in the emergency department. The didactic sessions in the emergency department are the following:

1. Registration techniques, consent forms, and medical record-keeping
2. Medical-legal problems
3. Triage and coordination of staff and methodology of consultation
4. Disaster planning and supplies
5. Disposition procedure and follow-up
6. Preparation for transfer, ambulance design, and training
7. Human dignity of the patient, ethics, and costs

Faculty

The faculty should have some common denominators. Those who lecture should be known to present their subject well, and they should be able to speak from recent experience; research and special interests should not be part of the didactic hour. All of this would seem to preclude professors! In fact a young vigorous faculty is recommended. They should be paid for their participation not to reward them but to make the interchange a formal responsibility. One potential problem is teacher fatigue. If the course is repeated at frequent intervals, it becomes more difficult to obtain lecturers. Preceptors should be called on to teach manipulative skills. Resident physicians and fellows welcome the opportunity and the honorarium.

In summary, the Pennsylvania Medical Society has prepared a 160-hour, 3-week program to help second-career physicians to evaluate and treat emergency patients during their first hour of contact. This course stresses manipulative skills, and 25% of the time is devoted to didactic presentations. If the program is successful, physician-students will return to their respective emergency rooms with the express purpose of developing emergency departments. Further, they should be better able to direct their own continuing education, for as Will Durant has said, "Education is a progressive discovery of our ignorance."

REFERENCES

[1] Bouzarth WF, Jones KB: "Second career" workshops. Phila Med 68:85, 1971

[2] Conference on Education of the Physician in Emergency Medical Care. Chicago, American Medical Association, July 2–11, 1973

[3] Goldfinger SE, Federman DD: Postgraduate education of community physicians. JAMA 206:2883, 1968

[4] Harless WG, Lucas NC, Cutler JA et al: Computer-assisted instruction in continuing medical education. J Med Educ 44:670, 1969

Ronald L. Krome

14

The Role of the Nursing Staff
in the Emergency Department

There are certain units within a hospital where the characteristics of the patient population necessitate nursing intervention that is distinct from the usual general floor services. Likewise, the constraints on certain task performances is not germaine in specialized units. Emergency departments are clearly clinical units with these latter characteristics. In our opinion, full-time emergency department nurses should enjoy a unique nurse-physician relationship in which the traditional responsibility of the nurse-to-nursing service (and only indirectly to the physician) is appropriately altered. We believe that the emergency department nurse should be responsible to the medical director of the emergency department for policies and procedures, recommendations with regard to advancement and promotion, salary recommendations, and ultimate assignment and supervision of tasks. Certainly, the emergency department director should relate appropriately to the nursing service with regard to the acquisition of appropriate personnel, but the full-time emergency department nurse should be allowed—even encouraged—to remain the "property" of this highly specialized area. The relationship is summarized in Figure 14.1. To foster and retain highly skilled personnel, the authors believe this schema to be appropriate and workable.

The task of defining the role of nurses in the emergency department might be considered by some as a heretical one for a physician to perform. There can be little doubt any longer, however, of its necessity, especially with the enormous pressure for change being applied to all the health-care professions by various external and internal forces. If we can assume that everyone exists in two spheres—as we see ourselves, and as others see us—then without ignoring the right of the nurse to determine her own role (as we see ourselves), the physician (as other see us) might also be allowed the privilege of making inputs into the development of role definition for the nurse.

As emergency medicine has come into the forefront of contemporary health care, so too has emergency nursing. Both are new specialty areas of practice. Nor should it be surprising that attention is being drawn to this area, especially with the burgeoning of the new types of allied health professionals that has occurred. Indeed, perhaps because of this latter influence, the nursing profession appears to be seeking to define new roles for itself or, as some think, redefining old ones.

MEDICAL MANPOWER

Of those factors that has added impetus to this role-definition task, one of the most pressing and influential is economic. There are, however,

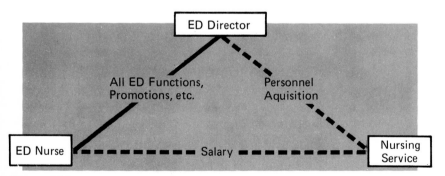

Figure 14.1
Relationship of the emergency department (ED) director to the ED nurse and nursing service.

other influences. The lack of sufficient medical manpower and/or maldistribution of physicians has led this country to look critically at the use of allied health professionals. The lack has also acted as a stimulus to the development of a myriad of new allied health professionals, each performing a specific health-care task. The medical profession has looked with new emphasis at nurses everywhere to see if they can play even more meaningful roles in contemporary health care, especially if the development of even more allied health professions is to be obviated. The press of nurses themselves to again gain their once close professional relationship with physicians has also stimulated role definition. Those who have spent their professional careers in the emergency department, like their physician counterparts, are seeking a new sense of self and a new meaning in their professional careers. The rapid development of the Emergency Department Nurses Association is a demonstration of this movement. In their desire to obtain the stature due them for the roles they already play, emergency department nurses are becoming more aggressive in role defining and are becoming recognized and active members of the emergency health care team.

ALLIED HEALTH PROFESSIONALS
TO DECREASE COSTS

To paraphrase an old cliché, the root of all change is money. This is especially so in the emergency department with its increasing caseload and, as some would have us believe, its increasing financial liability to the hospital. Health care is more costly, particularly with the rapid rise in salaries finally being afforded hospital employees. One way, perhaps, of decreasing costs is to use highly trained technical allied health scientists to perform those tasks not requiring a physician. In this way, the physician's time could be used more efficiently, thus enabling, we hope, fewer physicians to see more patients at less cost without compromising care.

It has been estimated[7] that a well-trained registered nurse, with support from other allied health professionals, can handle approximately 70–80% of the patients entering the emergency department because that percentage probably represents nonemergency patient visits. We already know that efficiency of the physician in the office is improved by using physician's assistants. Their presence enables the physician to see 30–40% more patients.[7] There can be little doubt, therefore, that the cost effectiveness of a physician in an emergency department can be improved when allied health professionals are utilized to perform technical tasks.

ROLE OF THE EMERGENCY DEPARTMENT NURSE

Since 70% of the American population does not live in large urban areas and since, in these areas, the initial evaluation of the patient in the emergency department frequently falls to the registered nurse, it is obvious that both the size of the hospital and the community served influence the role the nurse will play. Indeed, in these areas the emergency department nurse may not only be the first to see the patient, but may also have primary responsibility for patient care during the 15–30 min the physician may take to get to the hospital. Even in large urban areas, some emergency departments provide for 24-hour nurse coverage on-site, but not 24-hour physician coverage.[5] Thus the emergency nurse may be required to evaluate the patient in-depth and to initiate appropriate life-saving treatment.[8]

Perhaps nowhere else in contemporary medicine is the value of the physician/nurse team approach more obvious than in the emergency department,[2,9] and nowhere else is the nurse so vitally a part of the decision-making process.

In deciding what the role of the nurse in an emergency department should be, there are additional local determinants that should be considered. Their utilization may be influenced by, among other things, local hospital custom; state laws governing medical and/or nursing practice; the variety of emergency department patients; the physician coverage of the emergency department; the existing nursing staff coverage and the level of their training; and the relationship between the medical staff and the nursing staff.

Another factor that may influence the role the nurse will play is the availability of house staff and/or medical students. Many technical tasks that could and should be delegated to the nursing staff must also be mastered by the medical trainee as a part of his education. In those hospitals, therefore, where house staff and/or medical students are readily available and where they frequently and regularly participate in the provision of emergency health care, the role of the nurse on the team may be minimized.

Be that as it may, a determination of the technical skills the nurse should perform should be made, clearly defined, and written. Simple technical skills may be done by less highly trained personnel than the registered nurse (taking ECGs, drawing blood, etc.), even though they are considered part of the nursing staff. Which performance skills are to be done by which member of the nursing staff must be defined and codified in each hospital. Areas in which the staff may function without the direct (verbal or written) orders of the physician (*i.e.*, where the nurse can function independently) should also be defined.

Generally the emergency department nursing staff should take their overall direction from the physician-director. Direct supervision should, however, be done by nursing supervisory personnel. Even when the nurse can function without direct orders, some responsibility for nursing activity and level of function should be assumed or shared with the medical staff.

Policies and procedures governing the tasks performed and roles to be assumed by various personnel (medical and nonmedical) in the department should be written, distributed, and periodically reviewed and revised. In addition to routine nursing functions, the emergency department nurse must have the capacity to evaluate the level of the patient's problem and, within broad limits, initiate appropriate therapy.

The role that the emergency physician plays in the nurse's training consists of providing the basic knowledge and skills in the "medical" area over and beyond nursing knowledge. He should participate in the selection of nurses for the emergency department and then provide sufficient instruction so that their nursing skills can be expanded to enable them to function as the physician's "associate."[1] The supervision of inservice training and review of performance should also be under the leadership and general responsibility of the emergency physician, although directed by the nursing supervisor.

TRAINING OF THE EMERGENCY DEPARTMENT NURSE

Several authors have discussed the qualifications and training of the emergency department nurse.[1,3,8,9] All agree that emotional and intellectual maturity as well as a complete proficiency in basic nursing skills are "musts." In addition, training should probably include

1. Cardiopulmonary resuscitation, including defibrillation and use of cardiac drugs
2. Intravenous techniques, including a working knowledge of fluids and electrolytes
3. Inhalation therapy, including the use and abuse of respirators and ventilators, blood gases, and acid-base balance
4. Methods of obtaining and maintaining an airway; intubation
5. The initial management and complications of injuries to the extremities and injuries to the central nervous system
6. Wound care, wound management, sepsis
7. Pediatric, obstetric, and gynecologic emergencies, and their initial management
8. The differential diagnosis of the coma patient

9. Initial treatment and diagnosis of, among other things, hypoglycemia and respiratory failure
10. The indications for various x rays and/or laboratory studies
11. The use of the ECG and the interpretation of the cardiogram with specific emphasis on arrythmias
12. Resuscitation of the trauma patient
13. Indications for consultation and knowing from whom the consultation should be obtained

The emergency department nurse must have knowledge of current communication methods (two-way radio and telemetry) and an ability to use them, emergency transportation, and the value of treatment at the scene. The nurse must be willing to participate in emergency health care research and also be a "researcher."

We have described in some detail the educational needs of the emergency department nurse in order to assume the role as the physician's assistant. In addition to this role, there are others for the nurse to play in the emergency department that extend this primary nursing function. It should be obvious that we consider the most vital, most critical role—physician's assistant and independent nurse professional—the ability to function independent of the physician, assess the patient, and initiate therapy.

THE PATIENT'S ADVOCATE

The nurse in an emergency department can also function as the patient's advocate, expediting patient flow and calling to the attention of the physician those patients requiring his immediate care. By initiating therapy, such as ordering appropriate laboratory and x-ray studies, the emergency nurse protects the patient and expedites his care, while improving patient flow and enabling the physician to function more efficiently and effectively, utilizing his time to the patient's best advantage.

Follow-Up Care

In the provision of follow-up care, the emergency nurse can also act as a counselor to the patient and family to insure that the patient understands his treatment, current and continuing, and as a "follow-up" nurse. In a recent study, one emergency department used a registered nurse to insure proper follow-up care for emergency patients.[4] The nurse saw patients either in the office or in their homes until an adequate medical/social disposition was made. The follow-up nurse referred patients to the visiting nurses when indicated. In conjunction with the emergency physician, by independent review of x rays and laboratory work, the nurse was able to identify patients who should have been followed but weren't scheduled for follow-up by the physician. The follow-up nurse also made rounds with the medical staff and thus was able to participate in postemergency planning for the patient; in some cases, the nurse was able to expedite follow-up care by the early identification of a problem.

TRIAGE OFFICERS

Much has been written about the use of registered nurses as "triage officers."[6] It is sufficient to say that, when an emergency department has both a large number and a wide variety of cases, it is frequently necessary to establish priorities of treatment so that the most critically ill patient is seen first. The use of triage to insure that the critically injured are seen first and to keep nonemergent patients in areas of the department separate from critical patients can help increase the efficiency of the department and cut patient waiting time. At our hospital, we have trained practical nurses to perform this task. Other institutions have utilized ex-corpsmen or EMTs to do the same thing.

The wide variety of personnel utilized for triage points out the principle of distributing technical tasks, mixed with knowledge and initiative, to personnel specifically trained. As we have already noted, the determination of which tasks are performed by which specific allied health professional may vary from hospital to hospital and is dependent on those factors previously discussed. The principle of limiting the use of the most highly trained and most costly personnel to do the most complex tasks is the key to success.

Purely technical skills, requiring little or no judgment, can be done by nursing staff less highly trained than the registered nurse. Indeed, some simple tasks (starting I-Vs, drawing laboratory studies, doing ECGs) can be done under the supervision of the registered nurse. In this way, the registered nurse's time, as well as the physician's, is used more efficiently and effectively. Essentially, if we consider the physician as the general of the team, the registered nurse can be considered the captain and thus can assume the responsibility and authority that goes with a command position.

In summary, we have discussed those factors that must be considered in the role-definition task. Although we have stressed the role of the registered nurse and defined educational needs, we have also discussed the need for role definition for other allied health professionals in the emergency department. The importance of delegating technical tasks to the least costly personnel, while relegating the most complex tasks to the most highly trained (and most expensive) emergency department personnel should not only improve the efficiency of care but also make it less expensive in the long run. In this fashion, the time spent per patient by either the registered nurse or the physician can be used more effectively.

REFERENCES

[1] Anast GT: The physician's role in emergency department nurse education. Proceedings of Second Annual Meeting, University Association for Emergency Medical Services, Washington, May 12–13, 1972, pp. 49–51

[2] Fitts WT, Jr.: Men for the care of the injured: A crisis facing the 70s. Bull Am Coll Surg 55:9–17, 1970

[3] Hannas RR, Jr.: Staffing the emergency department. Hospitals 47: 83–86, 1973

[4] Jacobson S: The follow-up nurse in an emergency room setting. Proceedings of Second Annual Meeting, University Association for Emergency Medical Services, Washington, May 12–13, 1972, pp. 27–29

[5] Krome RL, Wilson RF, Schron SR: A study of emergency medical services in the Detroit metropolitan area. JACEP 2:177–182, 1973

[6] Platt FW, Turner W, Johnson R, Trimble C: Emergency triage by nurses. Proceedings of Second Annual Meeting, University Association for Emergency Medical Services, Washington, May 12–13, 1972, pp. 30–31

[7] Rittenbury MS: Training of emergency department personnel: Goals and levels. Proceedings of Second Annual Meeting, University Association for Emergency Medical Services, Washington, May 12–13, 1972, pp. 51–55

[8] Romano T: Trauma nursing in Illinois. Hospitals 47 (10), 1973

[9] The new E.R. nursing—Is it for you? R.N. 33(11):37–43, 1970

IV

Hospital Function
and Design

Charles F. Frey

15

The Emergency
Department—Function
Before Design

Often I am told while visiting the emergency department of a new hospital, "Our emergency department was obsolete the day it opened." Poorly designed physical facilities subject patients, physicians, and house officers to years of inconvenience, frustration, and sometimes grave risks. These problems can be avoided if the function of the hospital's emergency department is considered or anticipated in the design of its physical facilities. The function of an emergency department is defined by its area-wide responsibilities with regard to patient services, education, and research and will vary from institution to institution.

AREA-WIDE PLANNING OF EMERGENCY SERVICES

The necessity for area-wide planning of emergency health services is based on the need to improve the quality of care provided the acutely ill and injured and to reduce the costs of such care whenever possible.

The quality of emergency care may be expected to improve when, through area-wide planning, transportation of the acutely ill and injured is directed to those hospitals most capable of providing such care. Categorization of hospitals' ability to provide emergency health services, development of an ambulance transport system integrated by central dispatch, development of interhospital communications as well as communications between hospitals and ambulances, and development of training programs for EMTs are all steps in the area-wide planning of emergency health services.

Costs

Cost benefits to be realized from area-wide planning of emergency medical services may be anticipated through avoidance of duplication of costly facilities. The size of an emergency facility in the past has generally reflected the population that the hospital serves. Oftentimes more than one hospital serves the same population. In fact in the United States today there are many communities in which there is needless duplication of emergency services when the requirements for care of the acutely ill and injured are related to facilities available.

Facilities for the care of the acutely ill and injured include more than the emergency department. Likewise the costs of operating an emergency department around the clock are not accurately reflected in the budget for equipment and staff of the department. The emergency department is essentially a triage station in which the acutely ill and injured are channeled to the intensive care unit, the operating room, the coronary care unit, and other facilities in the hospital according to their needs. The staffing and facilities of these units to be available on a 24-hour basis are very expensive. Within a community, duplication of these services as well as those of the emergency department is an unnecessary cost of medical care.

Rise in Patient Visits

The spectacular rise in visits to emergency departments in the United States from 5 to 50 million visits in a period of 10 years does not mean that the incidence of acute illness and injury have increased correspondingly.[1,6,7] Visits from the nonemergent patient have shown a disproportionate increase. The reasons for the increase in emergency department visits by the nonemergent patient are multiple. They include decline in the number of family practitioners available on nights and weekends, mobility of the population, so that patients new to a community are unfamiliar with the family practice services available, increasing sophistication of the public regarding facilities necessary in the treatment of their illnesses, convenience, and cost.

Patient Triage

The emergency department designed for the care of the acutely ill and injured is an expensive facility. The cost of construction per square foot is high, and the equipment in the individual rooms of the unit is complex and expensive. Yet the majority of patients seen in such units are nonemergent patients with sore throats and a host of minor complaints, important to the individual, but not requiring elaborate or expensive facilities in their evaluation and treatment. These patients could be better triaged to outpatient or ambulatory care units whose facilities and cost of operations are considerably less than the emergency department. On an area-wide basis there should be a consolidation of emergency services provided the acutely ill and injured to avoid the unnecessary costs of duplicating expensive services. Transportation services should be organized and coordinated to deliver the acutely ill and injured only to designated hospitals. Concomitantly, there should be an expansion of evening and weekend clinics elsewhere to handle the increasing demands of the nonemergent patient. Proper utilization of available facilities will reduce costs and increase patient satisfaction.

Criteria for Evaluation of Hospitals

The categorization conference on hospitals' ability to provide emergency health services served a very useful purpose.[5] A set of objective criteria for evaluating a hospital's ability to provide emergency health services, which had wide acceptance by most of the major groups responsible for providing emergency health services, was developed and promulgated. These criteria will be helpful to comprehensive health planners in developing area-wide planning of emergency health services. They will also be helpful to hospital planners and designers of emergency departments who are now provided guidelines as to the services and programs that must be housed in a category 1, 2, 3, or 4 facility.[5]

The inhospital backup facilities for a category 1 emergency department are specialty staffing; emergency department staffed by physicians with more than 2 years of training; x ray, arteriography; blood bank; operating room and staff; intensive care unit; and coronary care unit.[5]

The mechanism of governance and regulation by which some hospitals would be upgraded and some excused from the emergency department business to run an evening and weekend clinic has not yet evolved. These decisions are probably best resolved by the hospitals within the same patient service regions, perhaps through or with the assistance of the appropriate area-wide or state emergency services health council. There is an urgent need for the A and B comprehensive and area-wide planning agencies in conjunction with state and regional emergency services councils to assist hospital planners by developing area-wide emergency health services plans for all states.

Transportation

Categorization and area-wide planning of emergency facilities will not solve any problems unless provision is made for a transportation system that will take the acutely ill and injured to the best emergency facility in the region. The transportation system must also take into consideration contingencies arising from the populations' incomplete understanding of categorization and area-wide planning of emergency services; *e.g.*, patients may present themselves or be brought by relatives and friends to hospitals without any emergency facility or one unsuitable for their needs or mistakenly to one of the evening or weekend medical clinics. Perhaps stationing some of the ambulances at those facilities without emergency capabilities would be one method of dealing with problems arising from the patients' inadequate understanding of the system.

The steps in area-wide planning of emergency services are

- Define geographic boundaries
- Survey hospital's ability to provide emergency care
- Categorize hospital's ability to provide emergency health services
- Coordination and designation of transport facilities and hospitals
- Provide care for the nonemergent patient
- Disaster planning

PATIENT SERVICES

The services rendered patients will vary from institution to institution depending on its categorization rating and its status of rank with regard to other hospitals in the regional plan. There are, however, general principles applicable to all categories of emergency facilities. The patient should receive prompt, courteous evaluation and treatment by the medical, nursing, and ancillary staff. The patient should be referred for follow-up care.

Registration Area

The emergency department facilities should be designed to provide a registration area permitting triage of the nonemergent patient to an ambulatory care facility (the ambulatory care facility could even be in another hospital or physically separate from the registration area) and the acutely ill and injured to the emergency department. The emergency department must be contiguous to the registration area.

Relationship to Other Clinical Areas

The emergency department facilities should be designed in consultation with all clinical departments and sections who will utilize these facilities to provide patient care. The director of emergency medical services and his committee representing all clinical specialties will be the final arbiter in the event of conflict. Cooperative efforts with area-wide planning agencies and other hospitals to avoid duplication of facilities should be initiated early in the planning stage. Methods and procedures for referral of all patients indigent and otherwise to provide continuity of care should be developed and promulgated.

Reception and Waiting Room

Often forgotten or included as an afterthought in the planning of an emergency department is the reception and patient waiting room adjacent to the registration area. This is a mistake in public relations by the hospital and medical profession. Studies indicate that 2.5 friends or relatives on the average visit a patient coming to the emergency department and that the number of visitors increases the lower the socioeconomic status of the patient.[4] Reception areas should be planned with the recognition that the emergency department is visited by patients from all walks of life in the community. The emergency department is a powerful public relations instrument; built well, it will engender good will. The reception area should be bright, cheerful, and comfortable; it should be of adequate size with provision for some privacy and diversion and adequate phone communication.

Treatment Area

The treatment area should be designed to provide not only optimal patient care for the acutely ill and injured but provide it in surroundings that will reduce the anxiety and tension of the patient and afford him reasonable privacy. Children and the nonemergent patients should not be exposed visually or audibly to the acutely ill and injured and the emotionally disturbed.

Inasmuch as possible the emergency department should be located close to those facilities on which it is dependent for services; *e.g.*, radiographic and laboratory facilities, operating room, blood bank, ambulance entrance, intensive and coronary care units, and specialty outpatient examining areas required by ophthalmology and oto-rhinolaryngology. The lighting of the emergency department should be color corrected. There should be a press and police room and space for ambulance personnel. Sleeping quarters should be provided for physicians and ambulance personnel, if stationed at the hospital, and for a business office.

Communications

Modern communications technology should be applied to emergency departments. There is a recognized need for radio communications between hospitals and between hospitals and ambulances. Not so well understood is the need for improved communication within the hospital between essential services and personnel needed during emergency and disaster situations. Additionally, there should be communication among all agencies involved in emergency medical services. Use should be made of electronic and television devices that will improve efficiency and permit a specialist in his office or home to participate in and review the management of patients seen in the emergency department. Examples of technology now available but virtually unknown to hospitals include the picture telephone for radiographic and ECG review and telephone dialing systems via magnetic tape that can automatically dial as many as 100 names in a matter of 2–3 min.

With increasing privacy provided patients in treatment areas, there will be a need for television monitoring and other electronic monitoring in every room of the emergency department.

The following list summarizes the facilities needed for patient services.

- Examining, treatment, shock, and specialty rooms
- Reception and registration areas

- Relationship to laboratory and radiographic facilities and blood bank
- Relationship to operating rooms, coronary care and intensive care units
- Communications systems and telemetry hospital and ambulance
- Sleeping quarters for physicians and ambulance personnel
- Psychiatric isolation
- Poison control centers
- Relationship to outpatient services
- Holding ward

EDUCATION

There is a woeful lack of structured educational and training programs in emergency medicine for medical students, house staff, postgraduate physicians, EMTs, nurses and other ancillary emergency personnel in the United States. Even in some major university centers, house staffs have been assigned to emergency work to provide a service often devoid of educational value. The need for emergency health service personnel is staggering. There were 60,000,000 visits in the United States during 1970 to more than 6,000 emergency departments, yet only 20% of emergency departments have physicians physically present in the department. Physicians themselves, most without training in emergency medicine, are filling an increasing proportion of this void. There are now estimated to be 5,000 physicians providing emergency services to hospitals as a full-time occupation. There are now approximately 350,000 ambulance drivers in the United States. For the most part ambulance personnel are untrained beyond an advanced Red Cross first-aid course, but demands for more sophisticated training programs are mounting. Emergency department nurses have formed a new specialty and are seeking training programs. Yet the educational needs of emergency medicine have gone largely unrecognized by university centers.[2]

Regional Programs

Not all hospitals could or should attempt to provide educational and training programs for emergency personnel. Educational programs no less than patient services in emergency medicine should be developed on a regional basis to avoid duplication of effort and facilities and staff. Training of medical students, house staff, and postgraduate physicians in emergency medicine should probably be confined within a state to

187

a few large academic centers having a category 1 and 2 rating.[5] Training of nurses, EMTs, and other ancillary personnel could be more decentralized in community hospitals and community colleges.

Decisions regarding the need for training programs at a particular hospital would depend on the population served and the availability of other training programs in the region.

Design of Educational Facilities

In the design of the physical plant of those hospitals committed to educational programs in emergency health services, conference rooms and appropriate audiovisual equipment should be included and are just as much an integral part of the mission of that hospital's emergency department as the patient service areas.

The increasingly recognized need of the EMT for sophisticated training in endotracheal intubation, I-V fluid therapy, relief of tension pneumothorax, cardiac monitoring, and defibrillation mean these personnel will be coming more and more into the hospital for part of their training. Classrooms must also be anticipated in the design of new emergency facilities. In the larger centers providing a complete educational program for all types of emergency personnel, space must be provided for a department of emergency medicine. These departments will have responsibility for educational programs, quality of patient care, and research into the delivery of emergency health services.

In summary, educational programs in emergency medicine should be provided for medical students; emergency department nurses; house staff in surgery, medicine, and pediatrics; residents in emergency medicine; EMTs; and postgraduate emergency physicians.

RESEARCH

At a time when the public is increasingly critical of the costs of medical care, it is ironic how little effort has been expended and how few published reports are available, even from academic centers, on the delivery of emergency health services in the United States.

There is a need for studying patient load, peak patient loads, population trends, staffing patterns, creative use of personnel, physician's assistants, patient flow, triage systems, transportation systems, the value of separate nursing services, innovative administrative and nursing systems, relationship of size of facilities to patient load, and how large a resuscitation room should be (square feet).

Patient Records

In a recent study I contacted eight hospitals, three of which were university connected and none of which could provide me with such basic information as, "What are the 50 most common problems seen in your emergency department annually?" This example points up the glaring deficiency of emergency department record systems in the United States. They are virtually useless for planning purposes. Emergency department records should be developed to identify existing problems, to point the way to needed improvements in patient care.

Records of care provided patients in the ambulance should be integrated with the emergency department and hospital records to make possible a comprehensive examination of the chain of care provided the acutely ill and injured in which weakness of any link might be detrimental to good patient care. Not only should information be collected regarding specific illness and injury, but enough should be collected to evaluate the efficiency of the whole system of emergency care. These records should be reviewed by a panel of physicians. They should be responsible for recommending changes to improve the care of the acutely ill and injured.

State- and Area-Wide Plans

Helpful to those responsible for designing a particular emergency department will be the development of state- and area-wide plans defining the responsibilities of each hospital's emergency department for patient care, education, and research. The areas in which research in emergency medicine is needed are:

1. Operation of the emergency department: patient load, peak patient loads, area population trends, staffing patterns, creative use of allied health personnel, patient flow, triage systems, transportation systems, distribution of space, space requirements, visitor loads, costs
2. Function of the emergency department within an area-wide system
3. Study of specific diseases

Nationally, specialists in hospital design should develop model emergency departments for different sizes of hospitals having a variety of educational, patient care, and research responsibilities. Availability of such models would be helpful to designers of emergency facilities. As the Committee on Trauma of the American College of Surgeons says,

"That existing emergency departments usually constitute the weakest and most neglected link in the chain of hospital care is beyond doubt. It is equally clear that the emergency departments of most general hospitals need renovation or replacement. Few persons responsible for these changes have any valid notion of what to plan or how to do it."[3]

SUMMARY

The function of an emergency department must be defined before it can be designed. The function of an emergency department is affected by its area-wide responsibilities with regard to patient services, education, and research and will vary from institution to institution. Hospital architects designing emergency departments will be aided by the early development of state and regional emergency services plans and models of emergency department plan for hospitals of different bed size, patient service, and educational and research responsibilities.

The emergency department planning function before design is (1) to define responsibilities of the emergency department with regard to patient care, education, and research and (2) to design facilities to meet the responsibilities of the emergency departments.

REFERENCES

[1] Canizaro PC: Management of the non-emergent patient. J Trauma 11: 544–551, 1971

[2] Frey CF: University Association for Emergency Medical Services, Charter meeting, opening remarks. J Trauma 11:541–542, 1971

[3] Guidelines for design and function of a hospital emergency department. Chicago, American College of Surgeons, Committee on Trauma, 1970

[4] Mangold K: personal communication

[5] Recommendations of the conference on the guidelines for the categorization of hospital emergency capabilities. Chicago, American Medical Association, 1971

[6] Research survey of hospitals: Inpatient and outpatient service units, 1969. Hospitals 44:499, 1970

[7] Walt AJ: The administration of the emergency room; of wicked step-mothers, ugly sisters, and academic Cinderellas. J Trauma 11:554–557, 1971

Karl G. Mangold

16

Policies and Procedures of the Department of Emergency Medicine

The authoritarian ring of the phrase "policies and procedures of the emergency department" is frequently lost the day after the survey team from the Joint Commission on Accreditation of Hospitals (JCAH) leaves the hospital premises. In the hectic, pressured time prior to hospital accreditation, a formal, rigid, and nonfunctional document is frequently produced to fulfill the standards of JCAH. Ideally, this manual should be continuously updated wherever appropriate and reviewed on an annual basis. However, the difficulty of documenting and commenting on all the contingencies within a complex area such as the emergency department usually results in neglect until just prior to JCAH examination.

The alternative to a rigid, formal policy and procedure manual is a practical, functional document that can be utilized on the spur of the moment and can be relied upon to provide clear, concise cookbook-type answers to day-to-day problems. The need for this type of manual is especially true in emergency departments that are unfortunately subjected to a high turnover rate of physicians, nurses, clerks, students, orderlies, etc.

DEFINITIONS

A policy is by definition, according to Webster, "wisdom in the management of affairs"; "management based on worldly wisdom"; and "a settled course adopted and followed by an institution."

An emergency department policy consequently should be a general statement that expresses management's policy. This policy must be general in that it should permit independent action by the emergency department personnel.

A procedure is by definition, according to Webster, "manner, or method of acting in a process or course of action"; "the continuation of a process or operation"; and "customary method of conducting business."

An emergency department procedure therefore is a specific statement that is much more definite than a policy. The procedure is a stepwise protocol on implementing emergency department policies.

REASON FOR EXISTENCE

The reason policy and procedure manuals exist is to insure conformity and consistency of acceptable standards and levels of practice within the emergency department. Additionally, in the real world, policy and procedure manuals exist because they are required by the JCAH.

The manual once in existence and approved should be totally accessible, in full view, and conducive to use. It should be concisely indexed and the information presented simply for total comprehension.

PHILOSOPHY

It is obviously impossible to delineate each and every emergency department situation. It is possible, however, and necessary to formulate policy and procedure for as many predictable situations as is possible and to specify plans of action for as many contingencies as seem appropriate. It is usual for the hospital legal counsel to be opposed to highly specific policies and procedures because of the legal axiom "to list is to limit."

192

ED—Policies and Procedures

The policy and procedure manual should be written by groups of people including representatives of the emergency department nursing staff, emergency department clerical and supporting staff, the hospital business personnel, the hospital and medical staff emergency committees, the practicing emergency physicians, and the hospital administration. Under no circumstances should an individual write the policy and procedure manual. All too frequently it happens that two people sit down 1 month prior to accreditation and "put the manual in order."

The emergency committee should coordinate the multiplicity of inputs from all appropriate committees of the medical staff, including the executive committee and the hospital administration, and the committee should review the manual prior to its submission for final approval by the board of directors or hospital governing board. Final approval by the board allegedly makes them responsible for its content and serves as "legal approval." It also serves as an educational experience for the hospital board of trustees.

SUPPORTING DOCUMENTS

Many feel that the courts have misapplied the decision of the so-called Darling case by holding the hospital board of trustees legally responsible for whatever happens within the hospital, including medical decisions made by independent practicing physicians. The emergency department manual must be corroborated and supported by appropriate materials, such as the hospital and medical staff bylaws, rules and regulations, consent manuals, emergency committee minutes, and those memos, notices, and executive committee minutes that apply to the day-to-day function of a department of emergency medicine.

STANDARDS

The accreditation manual for hospitals clearly states as a standard of emergency services the following: "Emergency patient care shall be guided by written policies and shall be supported by appropriate procedure manuals and reference material."[1] The accreditation manual continues, "there shall be written policies concerning the extent of treatment to be carried out in the emergency service. Such policies must be approved by the medical staff and by the hospital management. They should be reviewed periodically, revised as necessary, and dated to indicate the time of last review. Written procedures should be developed that are based upon these policies."

The standard clearly calls for two distinct policy and procedure requirements. The first requirement is policy and procedure as related to hospital administration. Examples of specific requirements are

> explicit directions as to location and storage of medications, supplies and special equipment; methods for around the clock procurement of equipment and drugs; . . . instructions relative to notification of the patient's personal physician and transmission of relevant reports; . . . plans for communication with police and local health authorities relative to accident victims and to patients whose condition, or its cause, is reportable, *e.g.,* persons having contagious disease or victims of suspected criminal acts; explanation of the disaster plan and how the emergency services are integrated into it.[1]

The second requirement involves policies and procedures related specifically to the medical staff and includes, for example, "medical staff obligation for emergency patient care; procedures that may not be performed in the emergency area, for example, those requiring general or major regional anesthesia which should be performed only in the surgical suite; procedures for early transfer of severely ill or injured patients to special treatment areas within the hospital, such as the surgical suite, the intensive care unit or the cardiac care unit, and, instructions to be given to the patient and/or family in regards to follow-up care."[1]

RESOURCE MATERIAL

The Division of Emergency Health Services of the U.S. Department of Health, Education, and Welfare in 1972 published a very useful guide entitled "Emergency Department Policy and Procedure Guidelines."[2] The pamphlet delineates 11 major divisions that may appropriately be included in the manual. The 11 divisions are

1. General and administrative policies
2. Organization and staffing of the emergency department
3. The medical staff
4. Legal considerations
5. Financial considerations
6. Patient management
7. Departmental relationships
8. Equipment, supplies, and drugs
9. Emergency situations
10. External relations
11. General hospital policies that affect the emergency department

Under each major division is a logical and comprehensive delineation of subcategories.

TRENDS

Perhaps the most important emphasis that will be required by the JCAH is the development of criteria for the evaluation of emergency medical care rendered to patients within the emergency department as well as an ongoing monthly audit of standards of medical practice within the emergency department. Particular attention should be paid to the following cases: DOAs (dead on arrival); DOA–DRA (dead on arrival-dead, resuscitation attempted); DIAs (death intradepartment); and D-24 hours-A (death occurring within 24 hours of admission from the emergency service).

Additional parameters of quality control utilization review and peer review of medical practice within the department of emergency medicine include the following.

1. A formalized chart review should be done by the emergency committee.
2. All patient complaints should be reviewed.
3. A copy of each and every emergency record of patients seen within the emergency department should be transmitted to the follow-up private physicians.
4. Official reading of all x rays by a radiologist within 24 hours. A report of this official interpretation should always be sent to both the private physician and the emergency physician. A mechanism of notifying and recalling patients who have had x rays misinterpreted must be clearly delineated.
5. Reports of laboratory results should always be sent to both the private physician and the emergency physician.
6. The official interpretation of ECGs should be rendered by the internist-cardiologist who simultaneously reviews the interpretation of the ECG by the emergency physician, and a report of the official interpretation again should be sent to both the private physician and the emergency physician.
7. Patients who are admitted to the hospital via the emergency department should have the care they received within the emergency department reviewed by the traditional audit committees. On reviewing inpatient records, the traditional departmental audit committee should begin the review with the care rendered within the emergency department.

8. A colleague-to-colleague feedback mechanism should be encouraged, so that follow-up physicians communicate mistakes, unusual occurrences, and follow-up results to the emergency physician.
9. A careful review of all transfer charts for safety of transfer and adherence to transfer protocol should occur.
10. Charts of patients who receive blood transfusions should be reviewed for indication of transfusion and consideration of component blood therapy.
11. The emergency records of the previous 24 hours should be reviewed daily by the on-duty morning emergency physician.
12. Protocol for retrospective and prospective studies should be established.
13. All charts of patients should be analyzed on a randomly selected day of the month.
14. Charts of patients seen by a particular physician on any given day should be randomly selected and analyzed in detail.
15. A formal step-by-step methodology should be set up for meaningful education by virtue of peer review, which would include (1) criteria development; (2) selection of cases within the diagnosis; (3) work sheet preparation; (4) case evaluation; (5) tabulation evaluation; and (6) presentation of reports.

The trend toward the JCAH requirement of detailed disease evaluation and review within the department of emergency medicine has become quite clear and should be heeded by those hospitals preparing or reviewing their department of emergency medicine's policy and procedure manual.

REFERENCES

[1] Accreditation manual for hospitals. Standard IV. Washington, Joint Commission on Accreditation of Hospitals, 1970, pp. 73–74

[2] Emergency department policy and procedure guidelines. Washington, U.S. Department of Health, Education, and Welfare, 1972

Milton N. Luria
John H. Morton

17

The Functions and Administration of a University Emergency Department

At the conclusion of World War II most hospitals were equipped with an emergency room which was often called, quite correctly, an accident room. Although occasional medical and pediatric problems were managed, most of the activities in the area were devoted to the treatment of minor trauma—lacerations, contusions, uncomplicated fractures, and other similar injuries.

In the years since World War II the emergency room has gradually enlarged and evolved into an emergency department. In the modern hospital this area must be equipped to manage a large number of patients with all types of medical, surgical, and psychological emergencies. In addition, the department is expected to supply primary health care for a number of people with less serious problems who can find no doctor or clinic to treat them.

197

Traditionally, the emergency room had a small permanent nursing staff, and physicians were available only on call. Frequently, the area was supplied with outmoded equipment inherited from other parts of the hospital. If there was a medical director at all, this position was assigned as a temporary burden to the most junior member of the surgical staff. Despite the growing complexity of the emergency department this approach still persists in many institutions, although it is clearly inappropriate. The emergency department is now a vital and complex part of the medical center; as such it deserves experienced medical leadership from a group of physicians who are able to devote significant amounts of time to the department.

A glance at the statistics from the Strong Memorial Hospital emergency department will show the dimensions of the problem. The number of patients treated in the emergency department was 15,418 in 1951 and 41,353 in 1961. By 1971 this number had jumped to 67,635; during this same year, there were 101,534 visits to the outpatient department and 92,239 office visits to physicians at the medical center, giving a ratio of roughly one emergency department visit for every three outpatient department or office visits.

Strong Memorial Hospital's emergency department is in reality a small hospital with approximately 45 beds in 24,000 sq ft of space. Facilities for diagnostic radiology are immediately adjacent to the department, and a room for a hospital-admitting officer is located within the emergency area. Between 150 and 250 new patients are seen each day, and 20 to 30 of them are admitted to the hospital. Over three-quarters of the patients are seen in the emergency department less than three times during the year, and 16% of those treated have no other contact with the hospital at any time. The unit is staffed by 15 house officers assigned full time with many more residents and attending physicians readily available for consultation or assistance. There are, in addition, 36 registered nurses, 5 licensed practical nurses, 17 nursing assistants, and 50 other employees. It has an annual budget of approximately $1,400,000 and, like many hospitals, it runs at a deficit, the loss amounting to approximately $480,000 annually.

There are five main aspects to the organization of the department: patient care; administration; public relations; education; and health care research.

PATIENT CARE

To deliver proper patient care the Strong Memorial Hospital emergency department is organized into three separate areas: an acute care area devoted to handling those patients with serious medical, surgical, or psychological problems; a nonurgent area, which, in part, supplies primary care to many patients who have no other source of medical attention; and an observation area to manage patients who require a short period of study before a reasonable medical disposition can be made.

Acute Care Area

The acute care area must be equipped with adequate staff and equipment to handle critical life-threatening problems. For instance, when a patient with a myocardial infarction reaches the department, he is not moved precipitously to the coronary intensive care unit. Rather, he is kept in the emergency department under ECG monitoring and close surveillance until his condition is stable. Since all the necessary equipment and medication for his management are available in the department, this initial stabilization permits a more orderly and safer movement to the intensive care area. A portable monitor-defibrillator accompanies the patient to make transfer safer. In a similar fashion it is rarely considered wise to rush an accident victim straight to the operating room. Unless uncontrollable hemorrhage is present, the patient profits by a period of resuscitation and rapid evaluation in the emergency department before operation is undertaken. Patients with acute psychological problems also require special quiet rooms furnished so that the patients may not injure themselves or others.

Nonurgent Care Area

Planning that will relieve the emergency department insofar as possible of the responsibility of providing primary care, a role for which it is ill equipped, is important. Providing some other facility that can deal promptly with at least a portion of the nonurgent patient load in the emergency department is one step that will allow the department to deal more properly with the genuine acute emergencies, which it is uniquely suited to treat.[1] Extending the hours for patient care in the hospital outpatient department and offices, with the inclusion of evening hours, affords one method of controlling the number of patients using the emergency department. Encouraging the development of neighborhood health centers and cooperating with those facilities once they are developed is another. If such centers develop without effective liaison and communication with the emergency department, neither area will be prepared to function as successfully as it should.

Another method of controlling patient entry into the emergency department is to provide an adequate crisis and health information telephone service maintained around the clock. A poison control center that offers advice about the management of ingestions has been a part of our emergency department for a number of years. Later, the department of psychiatry established a mental health answering service. More recently these two services have been combined, and general medical advice, an alcoholic information service, and a teen hotline have been added. These telephone services have now been combined into a single emergency service called Life Line. It is listed prominently in the Rochester, New York telephone directory and is widely used. Life Line is funded through community agencies. It works closely with physicians in the emergency department who provide necessary backup for the counselors. Since this service is available 24 hours a day, it answers the needs of many patients, thus lightening the emergency department load. Such a service, associated directly with an active emergency department, should become a standard health facility in any large community.

Observation Area†

The observation area is an important part of the department. Occasionally, it is not immediately clear what should be done for a patient, and a period of observation may solve the problem. Several illustrative examples will clarify the purpose of this area. A patient with chest pain who has normal enzyme studies and a normal ECG may warrant a few hours of cardiac monitoring to define whether or not a myocardial infarct is developing. A patient with abdominal pain may need a similar period of observation to allow the surgeon to decide whether or not to do an abdominal exploration for appendicitis. An individual with a minor drug overdose may be watched and released if rapid improvement occurs.

† Many physicians versed in emergency care disagree on whether an observation unit in the emergency department is an asset or liability in the case of the critically ill and injured. Some physicians view the emergency department as a triage station only. Following this philosophy, patients presenting problems in diagnosis or treatment involving more than 3–4 hours of effort before definitive resolutions might be expected would be promptly assigned and admitted to the appropriate inpatient service under this system. The physicians and staff of the emergency department would not be encumbered with patient-care responsibilities for more than brief periods until the patient was either discharged home or assigned to an appropriate inpatient service.

Other physicians believe it is the emergency department's responsibility to resolve diagnostic uncertainties and deal with such problems as drug overdoses and alcoholism in a definitive manner to minimize the disruption of inpatient services.

Either system can be made to work effectively if properly organized and staffed. The system most appropriate for a particular hospital will depend on the physical facilities of the emergency department, the number of emergency department visits and inpatient admissions from the emergency department, staffing available to oversee the care of patients in the observation unit, and the attitude and availability of inpatient staff to deal with emergent illness in addition to their elective patient-care responsibilities.

Some of the descriptions of the utilization of an observation unit might meet with vigorous dissent by some emergency care planners, both from the point of view of what is best for patient care and avoidance of medicolegal liabilities. For instance, the recommendation regarding the utilization of the observation unit for evaluation of patients with chest pain is a case in point. Unless the observation unit has complete monitoring facilities and available nurses completely trained in coronary care, many physicians would feel that patients with chest pain are best admitted and evaluated in the coronary care unit rather than in the emergency department. *Editor.*

ADMINISTRATION

In managing a large staff and a substantial budget it is obvious that administrative control is needed. A physician as director is in the best position to determine policy concerning medical matters. He requires the assistance of an individual experienced in business management to control financial problems. At Strong Memorial Hospital administrative matters are divided into five general categories: (1) organization; (2) personnel; (3) finance; (4) day-to-day policy; and (5) long-range planning.

Organization

Organization is controlled through an emergency department committee. Members of the committee, in addition to the director, include an internist, a pediatrician, a psychiatrist, a neurologist, a general surgeon, an orthopedic surgeon, a plastic surgeon, a urologist, an obstetrician-gynecologist, a diagnostic radiologist, a resident in training, two nurses, two social workers, and two administrators. This committee makes broad emergency department policy. Since the group is too large to be an effective administrative body, a small executive committee meets with the director each week to discuss and manage current problems. In addition, the executive committee supports and attends a bimonthly meeting in which the nurses and resident staff members working in the department air problems that have developed in their day-to-day work. The emergency department director is responsible directly to the medical director of the hospital and serves as a member of the committee that decides overall hospital policy.

No hospital can function properly without a current, carefully worked out disaster plan. Since the emergency department serves as the hub of hospital activities during a disaster, the plan at Strong Memorial Hospital is under the supervision of a committee chaired by a physician from the department. Periodic revision of the disaster plan is an important assignment handled by nurses and physicians involved in the work of the emergency department.

While every hospital is now required by the JCAH to have disaster plans, it is important to emphasize such plans are incomplete unless they are integrated into a regional system. This means that planning should include not only mutual assistance provisions and radio communication between hospitals, but also participation and coordination with police, fire, and ambulance services.

Personnel

Questions involving personnel are important in a department of this size. The medical director and the coordinator of nursing care work together to solve problems arising between physicians and nurses. Similarly, the medical director and the business administrator work together in relation to the nonprofessional people who play an important part in the smooth operation of the department.

Triage at Strong Memorial Hospital is done by a triage nurse who makes two fundamental decisions: she sends the patient either to the acute care or the nonurgent area, and she assigns the patient to a specific service. She is also able during clinical hours to send certain patients with dental or with gynecologic problems directly to the appropriate clinics. Once the nurse makes the assignment, the service receiving the patient is responsible for completing care or arranging consultation if further assistance is necessary. The triage nurse may order appropriate roentgenograms and laboratory studies before the patient is seen by a physician. She is supported by a resident who is in charge of the emergency department for the day. The resident in charge and the triage nurse decide periodically through the day and night the department's capability for receiving more patients. This information is transmitted by a two-way radio network that connects the five hospital emergency departments in the county with each other and with the major commercial and volunteer ambulance services. This city-wide system has been important in spreading the case load among the hospitals in the city.

Although the need arises infrequently, the resident in charge is empowered to shift house officers from one service to another temporarily when a backlog of patients develops and to request assistance from the inpatient services when even more manpower is required. A cooperative system of this type works well between physicians and nurses and between the different specialty services as long as the arrangement is supported and controlled by the emergency department committee.

Two personnel policies not common to all emergency departments are considered very important at Strong Memorial Hospital.

First, since there are over 20,000 Spanish-speaking citizens from Latin America living in the Rochester area, an interpreter with background in the field of health care has been added to the emergency department staff. The presence of an interpreter and of other bilingual employees supplemented by the use of bilingual signs throughout the department has permitted us to serve the Spanish-American community more effectively.

Second, there is active participation in emergency department affairs by the social service department. Four social workers are intimately involved in the work of the department, helping in placement of the elderly or infirm and assisting with difficult psychiatric problems. The importance of this work as part of adequate total health care for emergency department patients has grown increasingly evident. Although the hospital cannot assume the responsibility for curing all the social problems that plague its patients, it can and should attempt to ameliorate those difficulties that contribute to ill health. Particularly with elderly people the disintegration of a tenuous arrangement for care at home frequently leads to an emergency department visit and perhaps to a prolonged hospital stay. The social worker attempts, through available community agencies, to support and rebuild the home situation rapidly. This approach has been of immeasurable value in supporting the elderly and in reducing costly hospitalization.

Finance

Adequate financing for the emergency department is critical at Strong Memorial Hospital. Financial difficulties stem largely from two problems. First, this emergency department serves many patients who are covered by Medicaid and a large number of other individuals who are just above the Medicaid financial level. Over half our patients come from the two areas in the county with the lowest socioeconomic status, and patients with limited resources can ill afford to pay emergency department charges. Second, the local Blue Cross plan, the predominant health insurance agency in the area, does not cover most emergency department visits for nonsurgical conditions unless hospital admission is required. Since many lay people (and some physicians) are not aware of this distinction in coverage, patients may receive unexpected bills, which they are reluctant to pay.

No real solutions to the financial burden on the hospital created by the emergency department are in sight, but continued exploration of the problem with those interested in insurance planning and in prepayment programs is important. The other aspect of financing—making certain that funds are judiciously employed—is equally important.

Day-to-Day Policy

The emergency department committee has developed a detailed manual of policies and procedures. Interpreting these principles and making day-to-day decisions are the functions of the director and the executive committee. These seemingly humdrum tasks are essential if the department is to function efficiently. With any large group of people working closely together, points of friction are bound to occur. Knowing that someone is available to listen to and investigate problems when they do arise has an important positive effect on morale. Knowing that doctors, nurses, and administrators meet on a regular basis at frequent intervals to review departmental operations and plans is equally important.

Long-Range Planning

Long-range planning is a difficult but important aspect of emergency department administration. The department must relate to other areas in the hospital and to the community that it serves. What the department does and plans to do in the future affects the developmental needs of other hospital areas, such as the diagnostic radiology department, the outpatient department, and the operating room. It is important that no one area makes its plans without reference to what is being developed elsewhere in the hospital.

Communication with the general public is also important. The community must realize that an ever-increasing demand for emergency services may produce a situation so overloaded that it ceases to function efficiently. Fortunately, there are some current indications that these demands may be leveling off after rising for over 20 years.

PUBLIC RELATIONS

Communication with individuals and groups treated in the emergency department is an important function. In an area that cares for so many sick people each day it is not surprising that comments and complaints are received regularly from the public that is served.

Waiting

The basic philosophy of the emergency department is that the most critically ill or injured person will be treated first, while others wait, and this abandonment of the first-come, first-served principle does create a problem in public relations, since a number of individuals are kept waiting for long periods. Members of the department respond by letter or telephone to complaints about this policy and explain its rationale. Before the patient understands this principle, he is apt to believe that he is the victim of discrimination. Once it is understood that the same rules apply to all, that everyone waits while the patient with the most serious problem is helped, complaints usually disappear.

Cost

The other major complaint from the public concerns the cost of emergency department care. This care is not cheap, and almost half the patients treated have no third-party coverage to pay the bill. An effort must be made to help people realize why emergency care is expensive, but in view of the pressing financial problems the department encounters, it is vital that all legitimate charges be collected. As a corollary to the financial problem, the hospital works to obtain adequate support from health insurance, government, and charitable sources. It is essential for the public to realize that the emergency department cannot continue to function at a loss. Since the department is a vital community service, the community should provide it with an adequate financial base.

Communication

The emergency department does not exist in a vacuum. Since it is a part of the metropolitan area it serves, its staff should be aware of developments in the health field which may affect its role. For instance, a network of neighborhood health centers, partially funded by the federal government, began to function in Rochester in 1968. There are now four centers in operation. The first center to open treats a large number of children. When it opened, the pediatric case load in the Strong Memorial Hospital emergency department dropped more than 10% at a time when the medical, surgical, and psychiatric patient loads continued to rise. As additional centers opened, the number of patients treated by emergency departments within the community stabilized. The department should foresee changes of this type so that adequate adjustment in staffing patterns, in space requirements, and in supplies can be made.

The emergency department committee should communicate with many groups: ambulance companies, first-aid and rescue groups, regional planners, and law enforcement agencies, to name a few. When there is a local organization planning for emergency and disaster control, such as the Society for Total Emergency Programs (STEP) in the Rochester area, the department should be aware of its deliberations. Communication in both directions is needed; the community group should know of any changes within the emergency department, and the department should be informed of developments in its region.

The federal Health, Manpower, and Resource Development Act PL 93–641 has established some new relationships between agencies and organizations involved in planning and funding emergency health services. In short, this law establishes a State Health Coordinating Council that must approve or disapprove of all plans allocating health resources including emergency health services. This council, appointed by the governor, is to consist of 51% consumers and 49% producers.

Any committee or council developed to advise the State Health Coordinating Council must also be composed of 51% consumers and 49% producers. Formation of such a subcommittee appointed by the governor is usually desirable to focus attention of all committee members on EMS planning alone.

The federal statute also establishes a number of regions within each state, the number depending on the population and geography of the state.

Each region has a governing board. This board of the regional health systems agency (HSA) must also be composed of 51% consumers and 49% producers.

The State Health Coordinating Council is roughly comparable to the old CHP A agency and the regional EMS councils to the B agencies.

The role of the Health Department has been left undefined. A piece of model legislation for the state of Michigan that would include the Health Department in the EMS planning process is included in the Appendix (Senate Bill No. 987). A schematic interpretation of the planning process is shown in Figure 17.1.

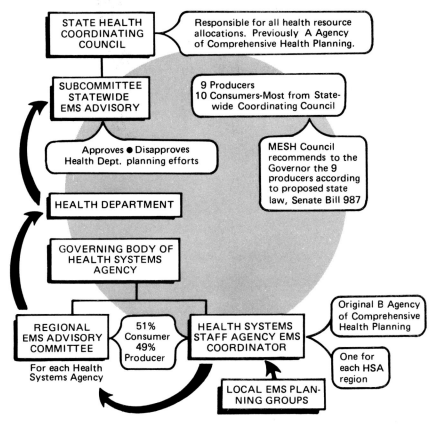

Figure 17.1
Planning process for emergency medical services (EMS) for eight Health Systems Agency (HSA) regions. The MESH Council is the Michigan Emergency Services Health Council.

Each of the eight HSA regions has a governing board. The governor's board rules over the HSA staff. All plans by federal law must go through both the State Health Coordinating Council and the governing body of the HSA.

The plans of local groups go to the staff of the HSA, a regional body, which reviews the plans. They are then sent to the regional EMS Advisory Committee, which is the advisor to the HSA staff. The regional EMS Advisory Committee, if it approves, sends the regional plans on to the Health Department. The Health Department then coordinates the regional EMS Advisory Committee's plans and sends them on to

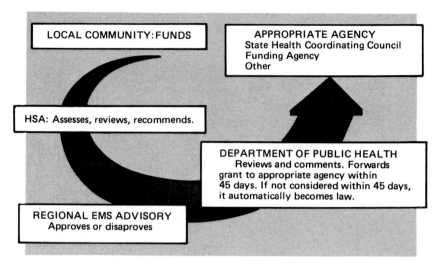

Figure 17.2
Funding process for emergency medical services.

the state-wide EMS Advisory Subcommittee. The subcommittee of the state-wide EMS Advisory Council is empowered to approve or disapprove all plans submitted by the Health Department.

The funding process is somewhat different from the planning process and is described in Figure 17.2.

CONCLUSIONS

The emergency department is not an area that is the exclusive domain of any one individual or any one specialty service; it is an area in which teamwork among physicians from disparate disciplines, nurses, social-service workers, and administrators is essential. Keeping such a system working as smoothly as possible and seeking to improve the health care that the department delivers are the two most important functions of the emergency department director and the committee with which the director works.

REFERENCES

[1] Carter JH: Planning and operation of the emergency room. Emergency-Room Care, (ed) C Eckert. Boston, Little, Brown & Co., 1967, pp. 1–17

James D. Mills

18

Triage

Triage is a French word (derived from the verb *trier,* to pick out) that means sorting, selecting, picking, culling, sifting, and/or choosing. An euphonious word that easily rolls off the tongue, it has been made into an English noun, verb, and adjective. Originally applied to the sorting of coffee beans, grades of coal, and the several components of a freight train, it came to denote the battlefield method of sorting out those casualties for whom scarce medical care might be helpful in restoring injured soldiers to duty.

In the last decade the word has been given a great deal of currency in America applied to the differentiation of patients presenting themselves to hospital emergency departments. It has been expanded to have a time sense in determining the degree of urgency of a given problem with regard to the order in which patients will be seen. In large medical establishments that have alternative facilities to the emergency department, triage is the technique for appropriate sorting.

In the case of multiple accident victims, triage begins not at the hospital, but at the accident scene. It then becomes a continuous process starting at the scene, in the transport vehicle, and within the hospital.

Effective triage may be graded according to usefulness: First, it has the least impact in routine operation of the well-staffed and well-designed emergency department that has a short waiting period for all patients; second, it becomes more important in the large, often under-staffed metropolitan hospital in which massive case loads result in routine waiting times up to 6 or more hours; and third, its paramount importance is in the effective care of disaster victims.

COMMUNITY HOSPITALS

A study of 40 community hospitals ranging from annual case loads of 15,000 to 150,000 patients deals primarily with the first usefulness category.[5] This is not to say that triage does not occur or that it is not important, but rather that it is intuitive, informal, and automatic. It is related to the judgment of the threat of the degree of illness or injury used to determine the order in which medical care will be given. This judgment begins with patients, their families, and friends who decide, wisely or not, whether they can properly deal with a medical problem. If they need outside help, will a phone call or appointment do? If not, should the hospital be used; and, if so, what is the appropriate mode of travel? Mercifully all these and more questions are answered by the routine decision-making processes with which most of us are equipped for daily living.

Once a patient is in the emergency receiving area, hospital personnel become legally and morally responsible for him. This responsibility must be discharged with competence and it is hoped with warmth for people whose complaints are so very trying for them and, at the same time, almost monotonously routine for health professionals.

When there is effectively no other place to send patients, then there can be no triage except as to priority. As Farquhar sees the problem:

> Patients who are in urgent need from major auto trauma, heart attacks, serious burns, etc., are given immediate attention. In our hospital, as in most others, every patient is seen initially by a nurse who takes the presenting complaint and is seen by a physician as well. There is no

referral to outpatient clinics. There is a limited referral to private physicians at their own request. These patients do not mirror the traditional concept of triage.[2]

Because it works, this is a nonsystem that does not cry out for reform. Skilled EMTs are very knowledgeable about urgency and have no difficulty conveying their impressions to emergency department staffs. Those arriving by ambulance are seen on arrival by nurses and physicians in sufficient detail to determine the need for additional immediate care and evaluation. When the EMT judgment is in error, it tends to be in the direction of overestimation of gravity, a situation that may raise the anxiety level but probably does no real harm to patients.

Most patients who present themselves to emergency departments are ambulatory and they are first seen by registration clerks and then by paid or voluntary helpers. This clerical pool makes all the obvious determinations of urgency, and the longer they do the work, in close communication with nursing and medical staff, the more judgments become obvious. They are easily taught to consult with nurses or physicians in doubtful cases. The most trying episodes are those daily ones in which the patient or his family is convinced the malady is much more urgent than the clerk envisions it. These episodes require skill to reflect concern for panic and confident assurance for angry epithets. There is no room for flip impertinence to patients whose own verbalization may be distorted by pain or anxiety.

LARGE METROPOLITAN HOSPITALS

In the large facility that must give service to large and often poor segments of the population, triage needs to be much more formalized. This facility, for whatever social reason, dispenses a wide variety of services but not necessarily with dispatch. Triage implies that there will be a receiving entity to which the several categories of patients may be sent. They may include the emergency area, which is the *raison d'être* of the facility; the appointment clinics; the around-the-clock pediatric clinic; the general medical clinic; the fracture clinic; the crisis intervention psychiatrist; the mental health clinic; the social service; and even the chaplain.

Sorting does not mean sloughing, so the triage officer must be a conscientious umpire calling the shots impartially and quickly in the patient's best interest. He must be above allegiance to any one hospital service when engaged in triage.

In the large emergency department typically burdened with a backlog of waiting patients, the system of triage must be organized to assure that everyone presenting himself for treatment is safely conducted through the screening, waiting, rescreening, and treatment process.

The individual responsible for this train of events may be a physician, nurse, or EMT. It is probably more important that he be well trained in the triage process than that he have a certain overall level of training. Unless stimulated, an individual becomes disenchanted with his work, to the detriment of patient care. For this reason and in the interest of the economic use of health professionals, it is useful to consider using people of various backgrounds specifically trained to perform triage.

Such a scheme is described by Larsen, employing clinical algorithms to provide control and simplification of the decision-making process for minimally trained personnel.[6] Using Red Cross volunteers and a collection of charts his group was able to perform effective sorting combined with the function of registration after a short orientation period. Skill and judgment are required for the design of the set of clinical algorithms "unambiguous step-by-step instructions for solving" a clinical problem.[8] Faithful adherence to this series of hard and fast rules substitutes very well for an intensive course in the recognition of serious medical problems. The volunteer makes no decision on medical matters, only judgments on which of two rules or alternative instructions are to be followed given the information the patient provides. The built-in, fail-safe mechanism is to make prompt referral to a physician when ambiguity is thought to exist.

Goodstein, Streiff, and Bragg made use of a *triage instrument* to better utilize the skills of aides in triage and to conserve physician time.[4] The instrument is an alphabetical index of 260 entries. Its function is to translate the patient's description of his reason for coming into a chief-complaint category, which will define the pre-physician workup the patient will receive. Although the entries span rather well the complaints usually made, provision is made for easy separation of conditions to an emergency category in the case of ambiguity in classification or inability to cooperate with the aide. Patients clearly needing immediate medical attention are identified through the emergency rules of the triage instrument included for appropriate items.

The health-care delivery system has the responsibility to optimize the triage process, and it falls to the emergency physician as a health-care specialist to be the patient advocate to improve the process.[1]

It will be readily granted that we need increased training and knowledge in medical care at all levels and improved facilities and equipment. What is not so well understood is the need for improvement in the triage process with improved communication from the time of discovery of the emergency, through control by the EMT, and to the emergency physician who has access to the rest of the health-care system. Planning for the triage system is an integral part of the total EMS system in every community and deserves scrutiny of local EMS councils.

All such planning should include built-in evaluation obligations. Reviews of cases that are a part of ongoing audits should include delays in providing care and any sequelae of that delay. They should also spotlight communication lapses having a deleterious effect on patient care.

DISASTER

The importance of triage is never greater than in a disaster situation. It is here that the battlefield horrors are paralleled. Only in disasters does one make the cold-blooded judgment that a dying patient may be hopeless and not worth the effort that would have to be diverted from more salvageable patients.

Disaster plans are discussed in chapters on "disaster preparedness." In all these plans, whether within hospitals, community-wide, or at disaster sites, the triage responsibility is of first importance. In every disaster we learn again how our retrospective vision exceeds our foresight. The varnish of civilization gives way to the animal needs for survival of self and loved ones. The best laid plans lack the needed flexibility. Journalists, morbid curiosity seekers, and concerned families tie up the needed phone lines and further crowd patient and waiting areas. Chaos gives way to order finally, and we critique our efforts with proper humility.

Reasonably, disaster response begins in the emergency department that in its daily work deals with many minor disasters and has its capability stretched with recurrent maximal case loads. We can exploit the only serendipity we find in disasters, which is that most disasters are small ones involving 5–15 casualties. Most properly staffed community hospitals can deal with this number without calling a formal disaster plan into effect. The advantages are that seasoned people know their capabilities, know what specific professional help is needed, and know how to get it. It is difficult but not impossible for one small team to provide life support for a number of patients simultaneously. Alternatively, there can be a plethora of physicians and surgeons each requiring nursing support and each acting out his traditional role as order-giving captain. When every order is stat, nothing is done stat, and confusion reigns.

The author witnessed a building collapse disaster in which radio newscasters described the horror, and the hospital council (representing 22 area hospitals) declared a disaster. One hospital received 16 physicians and surgeons and 13 casualties, one of whom was dead. Three patients were on litters, and nine were ambulatory. One other hospital became involved to a similar degree. A 19-year-old mason was a deathly gray. In 10 minutes he had blood drawn for typing and fluids running in each extremity, two of the infusions in cut downs. No one waited for vital signs; no nurse had the time to take them. A wet washcloth to the face revealed his ghastly color was due to cement dust. He was admitted with a fractured tibia. All the physicians had participated in prior disaster drills.

Care must be exercised to avoid an overresponse. The decision to implement a disaster plan should rest with those earliest aware of the dimensions of the problem and most experienced in dealing with emergencies. In the regular conduct of his work the physician in charge of the hospital emergency department is in close contact with public safety officers. He knows the capability of his facility and that of neighboring hospitals. On hand every hour of the day, he is well equipped to implement disaster plans when the need is present.

Sorting is the basic procedure in caring for large numbers of patients at one time.[7] Priorities of treatment are established with the objective of returning the largest number of casualties to productivity in the shortest possible time. It is in the mass casualty holocaust that the triage process reaches its highest potential. Since the classification of patients depends on diagnosis and prognosis, it is essential that triage officers have skill in making these determinations rapidly, coupled with the self-assurance that helps to make these awesome decisions acceptable. No triage is final, and the process is constantly updated to meet changing conditions in patients and changing resource availability. Physicians do not easily subordinate their usual decision-making authority to others, even in emergencies. The lines of authority must be clearly set out in the plan, and those to be involved thoroughly drilled in its implementation.

The treatment categories for triage which have been accepted through use and common consent are ambulatory treatment; immediate treatment; delayed treatment; and expectant treatment.

In emergency circumstances the length of time needed to carry out treatment is the determinant for categorization. It is not the severity of the condition, as would be the case in ordinary medical practice. Casualties with injuries requiring considerable treatment time, whether severe or not, must be placed in the expectant (delayed) category. Even though they may receive initial supportive therapy, their definitive treatment must be postponed.

To follow the battlefield analogy, a disaster requires a top commander with uncommon authority. Who he is must be settled locally, and this is part of the EMS council's planning obligation. Most important, he must be designated in advance, consideration being given to suitable alternates and standbys and assistants. All the public safety elements are involved and must know their roles. Assistants to the triage officers must be designated to keep the ongoing process of triage moving. It will be their duty to reclassify and also to render the only treatment allowable in the triage area (life-saving measures such as airway maintenance and hemorrhage control).

CATEGORY I. AMBULATORY TREATMENT

Most important numerically are those who can be treated in the ambulatory area and released. Because all resources are strained beyond their limits, patients will fall into this group who might receive inpatient hospital care in ordinary circumstances. The burden for appropriate follow-up instruction remains with those undertaking initial treatment. Patients should receive a record of medications received, the need for further care, and symptoms of untoward results. This information belongs on the emergency tag with a copy retained by the issuing facility.

CATEGORY II. IMMEDIATE TREATMENT

This is the designation given to the hospital area charged with the greatest treatment burden. The category should be used with caution so as not to overburden and render ineffective its important mission. Again, patients assigned to this group are those for whom early return to productive activity is a realistic possibility. The triage officer needs to be constantly informed of the capacity of this area. It is hoped that, once assigned to immediate treatment, a patient will actually be treated and not be shunted elsewhere except for unanticipated change in his diagnosis or prognosis. Patients may be grouped as appropriate into specialized divisions for immediate treatment according to services needed and available.

Sorting is a continuous process, and it is expected that patients will continue to arrive in the immediate treatment area as circumstances permit and as their original classifications are revised.

CATEGORY III. DELAYED TREATMENT

Patients for whom delay does not result in jeopardy to life belong in this group. Also, and a much harder choice to make, delayed treatment is assigned those for whom care is simply not yet available in light of the harsh, overriding consideration of potential for early return to productive function.

Patients who were in the hospital when the disaster began, who were not well enough to be sent home, but under newly imposed stress standards cannot now receive immediate treatment, are included in this category. Useful time can be invested in repeated evaluation of these patients to maximize the total hospital disaster effort.

CATEGORY IV. EXPECTANT TREATMENT

Necessary, but antithetic to ordinary medical precepts, this dismal area will be assigned those with poor prognosis. Included will be severely injured disaster victims, together with those whose underlying disabilities combined with new injuries decrease their prognostic outlook. They will receive attention to basic needs, including the relief of pain. They will not receive definitive treatment as long as the system is overwhelmed. Promotion to the other three categories will be the hope of this low priority group. When resifting occurs, it will be on the same principle of returning as many victims as possible to productive lives.

We are willing to admit that this odious category has, or has had, its place in effective triage for disasters. This is not to say we are pleased with it, that it is now necessary, or that alternate schemes are not now more applicable. Garb and Eng in "Disaster Handbook" present the history of "expectant group" in World War I and question its suitability in civilian disasters and even in subsequent wars.[3] In the light of surgical advances improved transportation within the nation as a whole, and establishment of specialized medical centers, they propose a more humane and progressive plan of casualty sorting:

Division I.   Minor injuries.
  A.   Cases to be handled in minor surgical operating rooms of hospitals.
  B.   Cases to receive preliminary first-aid and then to be transferred. Transportation may be by bus, train, or automobile.
Division II.   Patients requiring anti-shock treatment. These must be treated at once and cannot be transferred while still in shock.
Division III.   Serious injuries, requiring major surgery. (Most patients in division II would move to division III when out of shock.)
  A.   Injuries which require the most rapid emergency surgery.

B. Injuries which can wait from 6 to 12 hours for surgery without serious risk and who can receive such surgery at the hospital within the 12-hour period.

C. Injuries in which the risks of transferring are less than the risks of waiting more than 12 hours for surgery. These cases should be transferred promptly to other hospitals anywhere in the nation by the most appropriate method, including airplanes.

Division IV. Patients whose injuries are of such a nature as to require highly specialized equipment in order to have any chance of survival. These patients should be transferred by air to large university medical centers throughout the nation. Cases with more than 50% burns would fall into this category.

CONCLUSION

Sorting is important in all emergency situations. It is usually effective, though informal, in small community hospitals. When the backlog of patients waiting for treatment is considerable, it needs to be more structured. In developing triage persons, it is worth training nonprofessionals who can function under professional surveillance with high efficiency.

Planning for disaster response includes the designation of triage officers and alternates with authority. Actual disasters confound our most careful planning and require it be as flexible as possible.

REFERENCES

[1] An investigation and narration of the "triage" procedure. HSMHS Order No. PLD-9379-71-CM, East Lansing, Mich., American College of Emergency Physicians, 1971

[2] Farquhar JS: In Graves HB: ACEP surveys hospital triage system. JACEP 1(6):31-32, 1972

[3] Garb S, Eng E: Disaster handbook, 2nd ed. New York, Springer Publishing Co., Inc., 1969

[4] Goodstein L, Streiff K, Bragg FE: Evaluation of aide triage of ambulatory patients. Public Health Service Contract HSM 110169-264, Washington, U.S. Public Health Service

[5] Graves HB: ACEP surveys hospital triage system. JACEP 1(6):31-32, 1972

[6] Larsen KT et al: Triage: A logical algorithmic alternative to a non-system. JACEP 2: 1972

[7] PHS Publication No. 1071-C-5, Washington

[8] Sax HC, Jr. et al: Training of physician's assistants by a clinical algorithm system. New Engl J Med 288: 1973

V

Community Planning

Andrew C. Ruoff, III
Lionel L. Drage

19

State- and Area-Wide Planning of Emergency Health Services

The Emergency Medical Services Systems Act of 1973 represents the turning point in the development of meaningful emergency medical services in the United States. The initial impact of this act upon emergency medical programs in the United States will be the immediate dollar volume available to states and other political subdivisions for the systems development of EMS. Inherent in the writing of the act, however, is another benefit, a statement of guidelines that have been shown by those involved in the design and implementation of EMS systems to be reliable and valid measures of program success.

The purpose of this chapter is to coalesce the experience of those who have already developed EMS systems with the guidelines set forth in the EMS act of 1973.

PAST EMS PLANNING EFFORTS

State-wide and area-wide emergency medical plans and programs of the past have typically come into being through a process of evolution. These begin, in most cases, with the isolated activities of fractured provider groups. These groups are strongly represented by health-provider organizations and provide for little, if any, consumer representation. Their orientation and policy is directed toward special interests rather than broad-based program planning.

A subsequent phase of development has been the suggestion by some strong innovative personality within the state that the various organizations assemble themselves to channel their EMS activities toward common goals. Most initial planning committees are comprised of highly motivated, self-appointed individuals who are willing to participate in a process of constructive dialogue and confrontation to bring about appropriate emergency medical planning. Two primary activities of the initial committee have been to find a source of governmental authority and to obtain sufficient financial support to carry on their activities.

ORGANIZING A STATE EMS COUNCIL

The most effective line of authority for organizing a state emergency system is to obtain the support of the governor of the state and have him create by an executive order a state EMS council. This council should be broadly based and represent consumers as well as providers in all phases of emergency medicine. A typical list of such representation is the following: state medical association, state safety council, state bar association, state planning coordinator's office, state office of emergency services (civil defense), district EMS directors, and military.

Also, the state hospital association, regional medical program, state communications officer, state board of education, national guard, state division of health, state nurses association, and U.S. Parks Service may be represented.

The organized state EMS council should then seek a sponsoring organization, such as the state division of health, the Comprehensive Health Planning "A" agency, a strong health-provider organization (the state medical association or state hospital association) or the regional medical program of the area. Choice of the sponsoring agency may be determined by the capability of each organization, the special needs of the state, procedures for funding, or other state issues.

By priority, organization is most critical to the success of the state EMS plan. The first responsibility of the state EMS council is to define geopolitical areas in which district EMS councils can be formed. In many states, this procedure requires little more than dividing the state into areas that gives approximate equal population distribution. In other states, natural concentrations of population result from mountains, deserts, frozen tundra, islands, or other geographic formations. Some states are attempting to standardize district subdivisions; where these exist, the district EMS councils should be coterminus.

The state EMS council should appoint a staff specialist with sufficient authority and responsibility to assist in the establishment of the district EMS councils. This staff specialist would very likely be a professional health-care provider (MD) with close ties to the state division of health. Under his advisement, a district EMS chairman and vice-chairman can be appointed by joint action of the state medical association and the governor's office. The district chairman selected in this manner can be an effective coordinator and catalyst for the development of district EMS activities. Other potential council members are physicians, nurses, dentists, pharmacists, ambulance association, EMTs, health department, law enforcement (police, sheriffs, highway patrol), sheriff's posse, district officer of emergency services (civil defense), civil air patrol, military hospital administrators and councils, fire department, comprehensive health planning, educators, city council/county commissioners, television and radio stations, newspapers, telephone, electric, and gas companies, industry citizen organizations, and federal offices (parks services).

The active participation of the district councils in ongoing planning, implementation, and operation is the most critical aspect of any state EMS plan. To insure that the district chairmen understand their roles and responsibilities in the total state EMS program, they should serve as consultants to the state EMS council. In this manner, district and state EMS activities may be coordinated, and council members can be educated as to their role and duties. The following are possible objectives and activities of the district EMS councils.

1. Goals
   1.1 Improve EMS available in the district
   1.2 Educate the public on how to have access to the EMS system
   1.3 Provide financial support of this district EMS program in a fair and equitable manner
2. Objectives
   2.1 Organize the district EMS council
   2.2 Form appropriate committees of the council to assume responsibility of each EMS component

    2.3   Committees will complete a survey of the EMS components

    2.4   EMS Council will prepare a district EMS plan

3. Suggested Activities for District EMS Council

    3.1   Appoint district EMS chairman and vice-chairman

    3.2   Select council membership

    3.3   Write appointment letters

    3.4   Define council relationship to county health department

    3.5   Define council relationship to local EMS units

    3.6   Define council relationship to state EMS council

    3.7   Hold first meeting

    3.8   Establish meeting schedule

    3.9   Define objectives of each committee

    3.10 Appoint committees

Suggested activities for district standing committees are

1. Communications Committee

    1.1   Provide hospital-to-ambulance communications

    1.2   Provide hospital-to-hospital communications

    1.3   Provide single entry emergency phone number system (911)

    1.4   Provide central dispatch for all emergency vehicles

    1.5   Determine needs for telemetry

    1.6   Train communication personnel in use of system

    1.7   Public education

2. Ambulance Committee

    2.1   Survey of ambulance needs in district

    2.2   Provide ambulance service to all communities

    2.3   Provide ambulance equipment to meet minimum standards

    2.4   Standardize equipment with hospitals

    2.5   Determine EMT training needs

    2.6   Evaluate ambulance reports

3. Education Committee

    3.1   Provide self-help classes in high schools

    3.2   Provide EMT classes where needed

    3.3   Provide ambulance driver-training classes where needed

    3.4   Provide paramedic training classes

    3.5   Provide emergency-room nurse training classes

4. Hospital Emergency Room Committee

    4.1   Develop standards for emergency care based upon community need and capability of hospital

4.2 Site visit by district survey team regarding physical and staff requirements and medical procedures

4.3 Classification of hospital emergency room based upon survey

4.4 Based on survey data, determine deficiencies

4.5 Priorize needs derived from deficiency analysis

4.6 Implement program to correct deficiencies
  A. Provide training for all emergency room personnel to meet standards developed in 4.1
  B. Assist in proper utilization of existing equipment and acquisition of hardware to meet standards in 4.1

4.7 Staffing of hospital's emergency rooms

4.8 Provide highway signs with direction to hospital

BASELINE SURVEY

The next responsibility of the state EMS council is to survey the entire state regarding existing emergency medical services. Such a survey should include all 15 dimensions of an EMS system as stipulated in the Emergency Medical Services Act of 1973. Briefly, these are

1. The number and distribution of health professionals
2. Professional training and utilization of veterans
3. Communication
4. Transportation
5. Categorization of medical facilities
6. Patient referral patterns
7. Effective utilization of all agencies
8. Consumer representation
9. Policy regarding the ability to pay
10. Critical care and rehabilitation
11. Record-keeping
12. Public education
13. Evaluation
14. Disaster program
15. Reciprocity agreements

These 15 dimensions can be covered by conducting four basic surveys: manpower, transportation, facilities, and community and organization.

The first survey deals with manpower. The state must be surveyed to assess the number and distribution of health professionals, their EMS proficiency, and their previous training. This survey should include

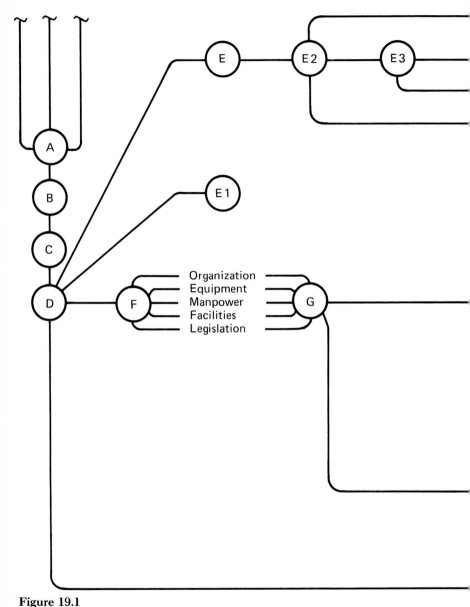

Figure 19.1
Overview of state EMS council activities. **A-B.** Form EMS ad-hoc committee. **B-C.** Obtain executive order to form state EMS council. **C-D.** Expand council membership. **D-E.** Obtain a sponsoring organization. **D-El.** Appoint executive secretary. **E2-L.** Locate new sponsoring organization. **E-E2.** Obtain staff support and council funding. **E2-E3.** Obtain feasibility and planning funding. **E3-**

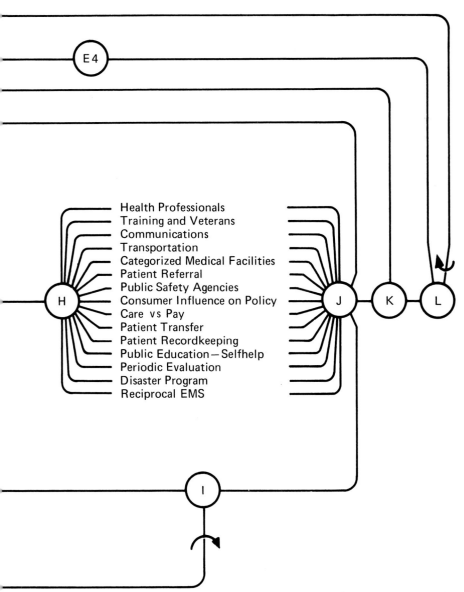

Health Professionals
Training and Veterans
Communications
Transportation
Categorized Medical Facilities
Patient Referral
Public Safety Agencies
Consumer Influence on Policy
Care vs Pay
Patient Transfer
Patient Recordkeeping
Public Education — Selfhelp
Periodic Evaluation
Disaster Program
Reciprocal EMS

E4. Obtain implementation funding. **E4-L.** Obtain operation funding. **D-F.** Organize council committees. **F-G.** Survey existing state-wide resources. **G-H.** Compile baseline data. **G-I.** Appoint district EMS chairman. **I-J.** Organize district councils. **I-D.** Appoint district chairman to state council. **H-J.** Complete a deficiency analysis of resources. **J-K.** Design EMS system. **K-L.** Implement EMS system. **L.** Operate EMS system.

ambulance attendants, paramedics, and Medex as well as the more traditional health-care providers such as nurses and physicians.

The second survey addresses transportation capabilities. Emergency transportation and evacuation vehicles include ground ambulances, planes, helicopters, and boats. Information should be obtained regarding vehicle operators, their communication capabilities, utilization, operating standards, record-keeping, and other pertinent points.

The third survey should cover all existing and potential EMS facilities. Traditionally, these would include the emergency room, critical care and rehabilitation units, and follow-up services. In addition, facilities that could be used during large-scale disasters should be studied. The facilities survey should gather information regarding the employed health professionals, their training, communication capabilities, the equipment available, patient referral patterns, the policy regarding the ability to pay, patient transfer, record-keeping, and disaster plans.

The fourth survey would be the community and organizational survey. The existence of EMS organizations in the state previously unknown to the council should be identified and requested to provide input to the state EMS council. In addition, communities should be surveyed to assess local interest in and awareness of available or potential emergency medical services. Local public education programs should also be identified.

The state council should conduct an investigation of the legal aspect of state-wide emergency medical services; this investigation could include a detailed study of existing laws, clarification or rulings from the state attorney general's office, and legislative enactment of laws necessary for the improvement of EMS. The latter activity should be carried on with the support and encouragement of the governor's office. Of particular concern would be laws relating to the Good Samaritan liabilities, EMT, paramedic or ambulance attendant certification, emergency vehicle standards, and other state laws directly affecting emergency medical activities.

To assist state EMS councils, several agencies have published guidelines or sample surveys. These sources are listed in the reference section at the end of this chapter. The data from all the surveys should be assembled in such a way as to provide the baseline study for the current status of the emergency medical services in an area. As a result of the studies, the committee will have specific and quantitative data with which to begin planning a state-wide EMS system.

The previous discussion of the initial activities of the state EMS council is graphically represented in Figure 19.1. It should be noted that this is an overview as opposed to a working GERT* (Graphic Evaluation and Review Technique) diagram. The example illustrates only 20 activities when, in actuality, 200 or more specific activities may be involved.

STANDING COMMITTEES OF THE EMS COUNCIL

The organization and activities described above are activities of the state EMS council as a whole or of select committees established for the specific purposes. The following discussion will define and describe for the reader the ongoing activity of the EMS council through its standing committees. The standing committees are communication, training, data collection, technical advisory, transportation, public information, and EMS medical facilities. Figure 19.2 diagramatically represents a state EMS council.

Communications Committee

The communications committee can begin to function by contacting outside consultants to help design and implement a communication program in each district. District hospitals should be able to communicate with all the ambulances within their service area and with other hospitals within the district. It is not critical or desirable to immediately develop a state-wide hospital-to-hospital radio network. The communications committee should be involved in planning and implementing a single entry phone number system and a single center by district for dispatching emergency vehicles. It is advisable that the high-density population areas within a state implement a system whereby all emergency services are coordinated and available through a single access number such as 911. Although it is not conceivable in the near future to make the 911 system available for all rural areas, a single number entry system can be had in most low-density population areas by using a standard seven-digit number. The communications committee should also be involved in determining the need for establishing emergency call boxes along highways and the emergency use of existing state communications systems.

* This is a network diagram for management planning and analysis showing the sequential relationship of activities necessary to achieve predetermined objectives.

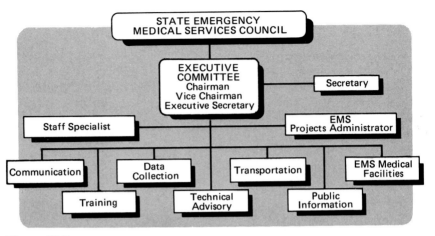

Figure 19.2
Organization of state EMS council.

Training Committee

The training committee should develop specific training programs to meet the needs indicated by the surveys. One example might be an EMT program. Although some states already provide EMT courses, these may need to be expanded, upgraded, or made available to law enforcement and fire department personnel. A more sophisticated program to upgrade the EMTs to advanced (paramedic) status may be needed. The paramedic activity is basically a method of extending physician capabilities in high-density population areas. Since frequent and continued use are the primary factors in the maintenance of paramedic skills, rural communities may be ill advised to expend energy and resources in the paramedic area. These would be better spent in Medex programs, as these personnel have the training to function throughout the total rural health-care delivery system. The training committee should often become involved in upgrading the standard of care available in emergency rooms by encouraging medical schools or professional societies to provide refresher courses for physicians and nurses. Such courses for nurses in rural areas have proved successful with high participation and interest.

Data Collection Committee

The data collection committee should be charged with continuing surveys as necessary and designing standard reporting mechanisms for information needed for ongoing planning and program evaluation. Most states currently have some designated organization for compiling state-wide health data. It is advisable that the data collection committee work closely with this organization. Initially, the committee will be involved in standardizing patient records for emergency vehicles and hospital emergency rooms and accident report forms. The records kept by the hospital emergency room should record not only the continuity of care provided for patients arriving by ambulances, but should also reflect the type of complaint and disposition of walk-in patients. Once these forms have been developed, pretested, and made operational state-wide, the committee should oversee the reporting activities and should continually work to improve and expand the data collected as needed.

Technical Advisory Committee

The technical advisory committee should provide for the standardization of hospital emergency room and ambulance equipment; this allows interchange between ambulance and the hospital emergency room equipment. This standardization of equipment can help to eliminate the current widespread practice of ambulance attendants waiting to retrieve their equipment and return to the dispatch center until the hospital medical staff has stabilized and moved the patient. With standardized equipment, a limited number of ambulances may be able to provide more continuous service to the population.

Transportation Committee

The transportation committee should be charged with upgrading existing emergency vehicles and/or acquiring such vehicles for areas that need them. It is recommended that the transportation committee follow the standards as established by the American College of Surgeons, National Academy of Sciences/National Research Council, and federal regulations governing ambulance design and equipment. Information on the need for acquiring ambulance equipment will have been made available by the initial emergency vehicle surveys. The transportation committee may also become involved in upgrading or establishing state-wide standards for emergency vehicles other than ground ambulances. In some states, the air evacuation or helicopter transport services are an important facet of EMS, and every attempt should be made to assure that care provided during transportation by these means is of the highest possible quality.

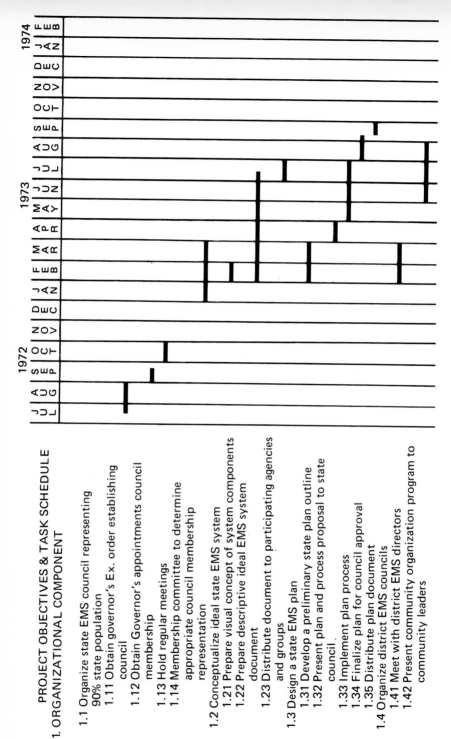

PROJECT OBJECTIVES & TASK SCHEDULE

1. ORGANIZATIONAL COMPONENT

1.1 Organize state EMS council representing 90% state population
1.11 Obtain governor's Ex. order establishing council
1.12 Obtain Governor's appointments council membership
1.13 Hold regular meetings
1.14 Membership committee to determine appropriate council membership representation
1.2 Conceptualize ideal state EMS system
1.21 Prepare visual concept of system components
1.22 Prepare descriptive ideal EMS system document
1.23 Distribute document to participating agencies and groups
1.3 Design a state EMS plan
1.31 Develop a preliminary state plan outline
1.32 Present plan and process proposal to state council
1.33 Implement plan process
1.34 Finalize plan for council approval
1.35 Distribute plan document
1.4 Organize district EMS councils
1.41 Meet with district EMS directors
1.42 Present community organization program to community leaders

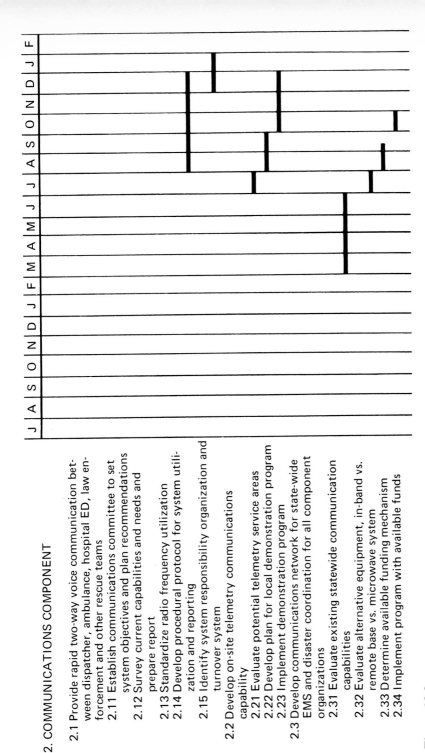

Figure 19.3
Network analysis of EMS activities utilizing the format of a GANT chart.

Public Information Committee

The public information committee should be charged with educating the public on how to access and utilize the emergency medical system. The committee also should participate in the improvement of first-aid and medical self-help programs. The consumer should be kept informed of the progress of the EMS plan and implementation phase. Each committee should, when appropriate, publicize its proposed activities as well as the benefits of any program improvements. For example, EMT and paramedic training have been sources of public interest and concern because national television programs have informed the public about these particular EMS activities. When consumers learn that paramedics may be functioning in their area, interest in EMS is increased, and the average consumer can relate to the system. Medical self-help or first-aid programs may also play a very important role in EMS for rural areas. These areas generally have fewer medical services, and consumers are located greater distances from the services. Therefore the ability of the average consumer to intervene properly until medical help can arrive is very important.

Medical Facilities Committee

The EMS medical facilities committee should be responsible for plans for upgrading emergency rooms and encouraging reciprocity agreements between EMS facilities. For these tasks, the committee should work in close cooperation with the state hospital association and the district EMS councils. The committee can aid the district councils in determining priorities for categorization of hospital emergency departments. Hospitals that do not provide emergency care should be encouraged to establish a routine referral pattern to other hospitals. The EMS medical facilities committee should also become involved in broadening the scope of special care units and trauma centers through the state. This process may involve establishing these units in areas that previously did not have them or encouraging hospitals to refer patients to nearby specialty centers. The committee should also assess community and individual facility disaster plans.

The activities and priorities of these seven committees will change over time as the needs of the state EMS system change and as new members are brought into the councils. The talents needed to perform tasks vary, and the transition to new tasks may not be anticipated or announced. By establishing an organizational structure with state governmental authority and strong local support, however, any new and unforeseen challenges can be met effectively and efficiently.

Funding

Continued funding is a vital component of a state EMS plan. Inasmuch as most states have a division of health responsible for the licensure of EMTs, paramedics, ambulances, nurses, hospitals, etc., and the gathering of vital statistics, it is logical to assume that they would be the sponsoring agent to fund and manage the state EMS system. The agency or department charged with the continuation of the EMS system need not be the one that sponsored the initial planning and implementation phases. The continuity in the change-over can be maintained by the governor's council on EMS.

DESIGNING THE EMS SYSTEM

With the information derived from the baseline survey and with the council divided into appropriate committees to handle the functional activities of the EMS program, the next responsibility is to begin designing the EMS system. Designing usually begins with a broad-based statement of the goal of the EMS system, such as "to significantly reduce the morbidity and mortality resulting from emergency conditions through the establishment of a comprehensive emergency system in the state of. . . ."

Setting the objectives to achieve the broadly stated goals becomes a more precise activity in that each specific component of the EMS system must set objectives that are realistic, will meet the emergency medical needs of the state, and are acceptable to the EMS council. The council should spend adequate time in designing these objectives as these will be used with matrixes of network analysis, GANT* chart studies, and budgets by objectives during the management phase.

MANAGEMENT OF THE EMS SYSTEM

In the establishment of a governor's EMS council, care should be taken by the council to keep it from resolving into "management by committee," a technique that is generally accepted as the least effective method of managing an organization. It is essential that the selection of a manager is done when a sponsoring organization is found. The director of the state EMS system should be appointed as the executive director of the EMS council. He should be from the sponsoring organization and represent the fiscal interests of that organization. Very little success can be anticipated in managing a state EMS system if the person

---

* Activities from the GERT diagram set in a format of a horizontal time grid.

chosen to manage it does not have the authority derived from these three simultaneous appointments.

The management activities of the director will guide the council in maintaining its businesslike procedures during all phases of the state EMS plan. Therefore it is desirable that this individual have a broad base of experience in the management of industrial systems.

Management by objectives has long been recognized as a process of managerial discipline that gives a high probability of success to management of a given operation. One of the primary responsibilities of the director of the EMS council should be to construct a network analysis chart that will relate all their activities in proper sequence so as to reach the objectives set by the council. The components of manpower, transportation, EMS facilities, organization, and EMS legislation are proper categories for the network analysis to begin and under which each of the necessary activities can be defined. Directors of emergency medical programs may well take the advice of those who have previously gone through the planning and implementation stages and be forewarned that the critical path in the network analysis of a state-wide EMS system is the organizational component that deals with the organization of the EMS council and functioning committees and the organization of the district EMS councils with their committees.

Without the availability of a network analysis such as GERT, EMS councils and state EMS directors often fall victim to the activity trap, little aware that the velocity of their EMS activities only indicates movement toward unknown goals. Most state EMS programs are only involved in 200–300 activities, and these can be drawn in a wall-chart format without the necessity of computerization. With this scratch-pad GERT approach to the network analysis and without using the sophistication of computerized times and critical paths, it is best to utilize the format of a GANT chart (Fig. 19.3) on which each of the objectives and the activities can be set in a time reference reflecting beginning and finishing dates.

Control over the cost is essential to the implementation of a state EMS plan. The executive secretary of the state EMS council should provide the council with a budget by objectives in which each of the major components of the EMS plan are categorized by a separate budget; that is the function of the network analysis chart and the GANT chart. The degree of sophistication that the council desires on this can be built in but budgeting by quarters or semiannually is adequate for most planning of EMS systems.

CONTINUED FUNDING

It was mentioned at the beginning of this chapter that state emergency medical systems frequently come about as a result of a process of evolution, and through these stages of evolution, it is not necessary that the same organization maintain its sponsorship. One of the most logical points to consider changing the sponsoring agent is the point at which the feasibility and implementation stages of the state EMS plan are completed, and functional responsibility and continued state funding is required.

SUMMARY

The organization and tasks of state and district EMS councils were discussed in this chapter. Particular emphasis was placed on establishing strong district EMS councils that have good leadership and that work closely with the state EMS council.

After the councils have been organized, the state EMS committee must gather baseline data relating to the 15 components of the system as outlined in the EMS act of 1973. These data can be obtained by four surveys: manpower, transportation, facilities, and community and organization. The information obtained in this manner may be used for planning and for evaluation.

Seven standing committees of a state EMS council were discussed individually with regard to their specific areas of concern and possible activities. The council as a whole is responsible for designing the statewide EMS system with overall goals and specific objectives.

Management of an ongoing EMS system can best be achieved by having the director of the state EMS system represent the sponsoring agency and serve as executive director of the EMS council. The system should be managed according to the objectives established by the EMS council. Activities should be charted by some method of network analysis. This, in conjunction with a GANT chart, will aid the council in directing its activities to the achievement of specific objectives and goals that will result in a functioning EMS system.

Allen P. Klippel

20

Organization of a Community Emergency Service: The St. Louis Experience

The results of the development of a well-established, well-integrated system for providing emergency medical care for the acutely ill and injured would mean the salvage of all potentially savable lives and the restoration to the best possible condition, physically and mentally, of all the victims of acute disease and injury. The component parts of an EMS system have been enumerated in the past.[13] In summary an EMS system has as its backbone a properly designed communication network incorporating both radio and land lines with interhospital, intrahospital, and hospital-to-ambulance capability as well as central dispatching of the vehicles.[10]

There needs to be coordination and communication with the other emergency services such as the police, fire and highway patrol, or sheriff's departments. A single telephone number must be developed for the public to use to summon help. Telephone call boxes must be provided not just in urban areas, but also along interstate highways. A campaign to educate the general public in how to achieve entry into the emergency medical system must be developed as well as educating all citizens in some of the fundamentals of first-aid. This latter is not only for their own use, but also so that further injury is not inflicted upon the ill or injured by well-meaning but erroneous rescue efforts. There is then an obligation to take the patient not necessarily to the closest hospital, but rather to the institution best qualified for the needed care. There is also an obligation to the acutely ill or injured patient as well as to the staff of a small rural or urban hospital to avoid delays by prearranging transfers to hospitals with better emergency facilities if a patient is found to need more sophisticated care than can be provided at the first institution. All ambulance personnel must be adequately trained to provide a professional type of patient care and handling.[15]

If it is true that the component parts of a good EMS system are so well known, why are these appropriate, categorized, coordinated efforts not fully and completely developed in every area of the United States? Opposition to these golden ideals should be a little like opposing motherhood and apple pie. How is it that a system for emergency medical care isn't available in every area, rural and urban, of our society?

It is tempting to review the parameters of a complete emergency medical system and then point to an illustrative location such as Jacksonville, Florida.[11] But, to understand why better EMS systems are not available, consider the St. Louis area and the efforts that have been expended there. The St. Louis Bi-State area covers four counties in the State of Missouri and three in the State of Illinois plus the City of St. Louis, which is its own county. In this area, there is one major city and approximately 110 minor cities with political "fiefdoms" and antagonisms that are at least 100 years old.

COMMUNITY INVOLVEMENT

It can safely be said in retrospect that if we had approached the local problems with some better understanding of the concerns of other groups, such as the hospital administrators or ambulance services, we might have made more progress to date than we have. From the Jungfrau pinnacle of a university, it is treacherously easy to pontificate, and an academic position can lend weight to comments to the local press.

If there is any one suggestion that can be made from our experience that may help other communities in the development of a system for emergency medical service, let it be this. Early on, involve every one in the community who is a provider of health and emergency care in a citizens council and include in that same council every interested citizen, including the news media. There is a very strong temptation to avoid the delays and arguments that occur when you deal with uninformed vested interests. It appears to be much quicker to design a regional EMS system and then try to beat the providers until they fall into line. Unless you have legal authority, as Boyd[3] did in Illinois, don't fall into this trap; we did.

Let it be emphasized again, that it will be time well spent to work with the providers and recipients of emergency medical services and curry their favor for any proposals and programs that may be envisioned. You may also find that some of your own preconceived ideas will change at the same time. It can safely be said that we made most of the mistakes that could have been made, and most of these mistakes were due to our desire to implement the system quickly. On the positive side, considerable progress has been made, and it is a lot safer to have an accident or acute illness in the St. Louis Bi-State area than it was a year or 2 ago, but very much remains to be done.

It has been suggested that what is needed in every community is a missionary.[12] It is hoped that the missionary will be a physician who, being totally committed to concerns about the deficiencies of care in his community, will be able to corner the mayor and the other interested people in the area and be able to form a citizens committee. This committee in turn would have the authority, since they were composed of not only public officials but also influencial citizens, to see that progress would be made to develop an EMS system and also secure the needed funds.[7]

TIMING

The design of the EMS program must be done in advance by knowledgeable people, but frequently it is difficult to get it going until something happens. Certainly the time to organize for emergency medicine is not when you are looking at wrecked, dislocated houses with howling people inside; nor is it propitious to begin the study of the parameters in providing emergency care coincidental with the extrication of multiple unconcious people from a building where an ammonia-charged refrigeration line has ruptured.

As a matter of fact the time for developing the mechanisms needed to handle even one white-faced, clammy citizen, whose car has fallen off a jack and smashed his leg, is days, weeks, and months before the event. The old adage "if you take care of the pennies the dollars will take care of themselves" is equally applicable to any consideration of how to develop an organized community EMS. If the EMS program is designated to handle the day-to-day medical and surgical emergencies in appropriate fashion, then the expectation can be held that the system will encompass the most malevolent vicissitudes that can be visited upon any of the citizens in any area.

As was said, the component parts of a system to deliver emergency medical service are known, and they had been known in the St. Louis area equally but to no great avail, despite the efforts of the local Committee on Trauma of the American College of Surgeons. Station wagons and police cruisers were being used for most emergency ambulance trips. There were virtually no radio communications. What private ambulance services that were available were used for transfers with untrained personnel in converted hearses. Things were about as bad as they could be in terms of emergency medical care.

There is nothing more likely to focus attention on EMS than a "good" emergency. It seems a little sorry that the electorate needs to be shocked into action, but a review of the development of EMS systems indicates that many really got started after some acute local problem or tragedy. It would be helpful to have the mayor or a friend of his run over by a truck and subsequently be mishandled. This is the sort of event that can be thoroughly covered by the local press, and a similar event did happen in Kansas City, Missouri. There a prominent physician with acute chest pain and a friend of the mayor, also a physician, waited for an ambulance for what must have seemed interminable hours. The subsequent findings that he had no coronary occlusion was a happy "coda" to the event. The deficiencies had been spotlighted, and efforts to correct this situation were started.

THE ST. LOUIS TORNADO

In the St. Louis area the catalyst was a tornado (1967) that skipped through the area touching down at multiple points. The tornado first became known to the local authorities when a message was received by a police dispatcher that there was a house in the middle of a major street, and the poor befuddled patrol officer wanted to know just what the hell he was supposed to do. This is not to say that immediately following the tornado the pieces of the puzzle fell smoothly into position, but one of the newspapers had found a "cause célèbre." Fine, now we had a well-publicized opportunity to illustrate our deficiencies, so let me detail for you our experiences and why we only inch forward today in the St. Louis area.

Lack of Communications

Let us begin with communications. During the St. Louis tornado, there were no radio communications between the hospitals, hospitals and ambulances, or, as a matter of fact, even between the multiple police departments in the area and anybody else. The first ambulance on the scene where most of the casualties were extricated was told to go to one hospital; as a result, every ambulance followed the first one with monotonous regularity so that this hospital received 150 casualties, and another hospital, two blocks away, received 10.

A significant finding at the time of the tornado was that, in addition to their being no hospital-to-ambulance communications or any other radio communications, telephone communications were very poor. Many physicians of the various hospitals in the area tried to call their hospital by telephone to see if they were needed. Distraught people called to ask about relatives. Reporters and the curious called for news. When the telephone circuits became overloaded the switchboards simply and automatically shut down to protect the equipment from the overload. Some telephone lines had also been knocked out by the wind. Communications of all sorts were probably the most glaring defect pointed up by the storm.

EMS COMMITTEE

As a first step, the medical societies in the St. Louis area appointed men to an EMS committee. The Emergency Medical Services Committee of the two medical societies then were incorporated into the local Committee on Trauma of the American College of Surgeons. Representatives from this joint committee sat down with knowledgeable people from the commercial communications providers and some television and radio people to begin to learn what a system for emergency communications should be.

A plan was developed that seemed mostly to involve hospitals, so this was presented to the Metropolitan Hospital Association with the suggestion the time was ripe to get moving. Of this nothing was heard for many months, and then suddenly the executive secretary of the Metropolitan Hospital Association called a press conference and announced that the area hospital administrators had discovered that there were deficiencies in communications in past disaster situations and that they were now going to develop a system of interhospital communication. The hospital association appointed a committee that traveled down the same road and met with radio providers and communication personnel and designed essentially an identical plan for interhospital communication. Eventually, contracts were let and the equipment installation begun. An unfortunate delay occurred just prior to inaugurating the system when one of the major regional hospitals had its transmitter and receiver stolen. To speed things along, just before the theft, a fight developed between the Board of Aldermen and the manufacturer of the equipment over another unrelated purchase. The aldermen would purchase nothing from this company until the problem was resolved. Six months passed with this impasse, then a compromise was found, and the replacement equipment was ordered. Since manufacturers make radios only after the order is placed, another 4-month delay ensued before the network was completed.

MODEL AMBULANCE ORDINANCE

Meanwhile the Model Ambulance Ordinance of the National Safety Council was proposed to both the city and county governments. Hearings were held in both areas by the various committees of government, and time and again it was necessary to explain that a sleek hearse-type ambulance driven at high speed by an untrained cowboy was not what was meant by emergency care and transportation. These prolonged efforts were rewarded in the next 6 months by the St. Louis County Council adopting the model ordinance, and a few months after that the Board of Aldermen of the City of St. Louis adopted almost an identical piece of legislation. Immediately the private ambulance operators in the county, largely operated out of funeral homes, announced that they would be delighted to work with the law, but if anybody got too sticky about it they would be forced to quit the business all together. The hospital administration of St. Louis County, being something less than stout-hearted, became something less than strict in the enforcement of the provisions of the ordinance regarding the training of ambulance personnel and the equipment carried on their vehicles. The city government, having enacted the ordinance, immediately was given a ruling by the attorney for the city that this did not apply to governmental units, thus excluding the vehicles of the police and hospital division. In all fairness to the government of the City of St. Louis, it should be pointed out that the city suffers from a deteriorating tax base, a malady common to all large metropolitan cities; in addition, the City of St. Louis had divorced itself from St. Louis County in 1879 over some forgotten squabble. Thus the city had only its dwindling resources to finance any new services.

Ambulance Service Before Passage of Ordinance

Ambulance service has been available as a municipal function of the City of St. Louis continuously since 1867, and even as far back as 1849 there were horse-drawn ambulances provided that took the victims of the cholera epidemic to several different hospitals. These ambulances were dispursed in three locations of the city, and this may well represent the origin of the oldest ambulance service in the United States, but antiquity guarantees nothing about ability or efficiency. The ambulance service in the City of St. Louis had deteriorated to become only a taxi service taking patients to and from the clinics at the municipal hospitals. This situation had developed during World War II, when personnel were in short supply, and in the name of efficiency the police department cruising patrols were called "dual purpose" and used to transport the ill and injured as well as drunks and malfeasants. The hospital commissioner of the time was looking to save money, and his medical advisors seconded this effort with such statements as, "Don't mess with patients, bring them to the hospital where real doctors can provide proper care. We don't need any overgrown Boy Scouts running around." At that point in time only an eighth-grade education was required for an ambulance driver in the happy hope he could at least read the street signs to locate his destination. If the ambulance had carried an attendant, which it didn't, the latter was spared this stringent educational requirement. The emergency patient was usually left to the untender mercy of the police who dumped the victim on a canvas stretcher, which wasn't even fastened down, and no one rode in the back of the vehicle. Speed was the only factor even remotely in his favor. The paddy wagons' operators didn't even carry a Band-Aid.

Ambulance Service After Passage of Ordinance

The new ambulance ordinance could not change anything, since it was ruled that it did not apply to the police or hospital divisions. It was readily apparent that having the new ambulance ordinance was leading us nowhere. For various reasons the authorities were not going to enforce the laws, and therefore they were useless. A different tact by the Emergency Medical Services Committee was next considered. We would go and work with part of the providers as a beginning. The need for training in the city and county was obvious, and a 40-hour course prescribed by the Academy of Orthopedic Surgeons[8] was offered to all ambulance personnel. Some of the municipal services sent their men, but the private ambulance operators lacked enthusiasm even for this minimal training; interest was low until the county government finally responded to some pushing and demanded the training as a requirement for payment for ambulance services provided to the indigent. Then there was considerable opposition to carrying even the minimal equipment suggested by the "essential equipment list" of the American College of Surgeons.[6] About this time, however, the State of Missouri began to provide fully equipped ambulances for fire districts under the U.S. Department of Transportation (USDOT) Highway Safety Program, with training provided. As fire service ambulance districts developed in St. Louis County, the enthusiasm of the private ambulance operators increased materially, for they began to see that the time would not be long in coming before they either shaped up or were shipped out. They all pleaded incipient poverty but fought to stay in the business. Still the men of the private county ambulance services were sent for training only as long as it was provided at night on their time off.

It takes money to run an emergency ambulance service, as the directors of the fire districts found out, and additional tax money was needed to support the new services. To get the taxes passed the voters were assured that an ambulance would be supplied anytime, day or night, at no charge. An ambulance could be called for any medical problems or injuries great or small, and the victim could be taken to any hospital. Fire chiefs now found their ambulances being used as taxis not only in their city but also throughout the metropolitan area. Since no charge was made for the service it was much cheaper to call for an ambulance even for a smashed finger than to pay a taxi.

A good number of patients delivered to County Hospital with claims of terrible sickness walked through the emergency department and over to the clinics for a regularly scheduled visit. In some communities the elected officials seized on the political favors of the ambulance service, and on more than one occasion an ambulance arrived at the supposed scene of an acute medical emergency to be greeted by the victim walking out of the house carrying his suitcase and announcing that he was expected to go to such and such a hospital. These occurrences should have been bad enough, but on many occasions the ambulance was dispatched to the same hospital to bring the patient, now recovered, back again.

Again the peculiar political situation of the St. Louis metropolitan area was working against any unified approach. The St. Louis County government composed of an executive with a representative council has a great deal of moral authority, but the only political clout it has is to pass amendments to the charter of the county, and these amendments must be supported by two thirds of the residents of the entire county. Most of the electorate seems to fear super-government and the county supervisor would not instigate any legislation unless it was certain of passage. So no ambulance regulations were issued. Since the various fire districts and their ambulances were and are autonomous, no coordination could be obtained. A crazy guilt as a result of ambulance service was only one small expression of the public's desire to preserve their individual prerogatives, probably to their individual dangers. The man who lived in a community with an ambulance service saw no need for county regulation, forgetting he passed daily through six or more villages with or without good or bad ambulance services every day to and from work.

Funds for Service

While the county was ineffectively thrashing around with this problem, the City of St. Louis, since it was obviously a depressed area with high unemployment, was made the recipient of federal funds under the Emergency Employment Act. These funds could be used to employ the unemployed in activities for the benefit of the area, and the ambulance service was to be one of the recipients. Some of the clamor generated by the newspapers was beginning to pay off.

Four ambulances were obtained from the State of Missouri and USDOT Highway Safety Funds and additional men were hired to staff these as well as the older ambulances using the Emergency Employment Act money. All the hospital division ambulance activities in St. Louis for 4 days were completely stopped, and the entire company of men including the dispatchers were given an intensive period of instruction. On the fifth day at 7:00 A.M., the new service was inaugurated. The clinic runs would have to continue, but they had become subservient to the demands of the new emergency ambulance service. The St. Louis police department was informed that, since there was now a good ambulance service, they would cease and desist in patient transport. The reaction of the police officials was enthusiastic, and seemingly they were delighted to have somebody relieve them of the responsibility of transporting the injured, but the actions of the policeman on the street were largely unaltered. The operator of the cruising paddy wagon or squad car refused to admit that the ambulance could be summoned and arrive within a short period of time. The "man" on the street now had to ask for help from another service, and apparently he felt his image was threatened.

At the time of the takeover of the emergency ambulance services, the police department was making 81% of the runs and the hospital ambulance 19%. Since the police department radio operations were on a different frequency from the ambulances, there was no way of knowing when an ambulance was needed until a call was placed directly to the dispatcher; it was contended that calling for an ambulance would mean long delays for the patient. This problem was finally resolved by ambulance representatives sitting in the dispatching center of the police department smiling happily at the head dispatcher and monitoring the calls, so that when an ambulance was needed an ambulance was called instead of the cruiser. Even so, this procedure did not completely resolve the problem, because the cruisers in the area could hear the police calls and dispatch themselves to offer assistance; if they arrived before the ambulance, they hurried to try to load the victim in the cruiser, although the ambulance was frequently in sight and descending upon them rapidly. This behavior led to some sharp discussions between the police and the ambulance personnel held in the middle of the city streets to the amazement of the patient and spectators. Increasing demands upon the police department from the criminal element gradually resolved that problem, however, and the more conscientious of the police have realized that the trained ambulance personnel provide a much superior level of care. After 2 years of operation, the police are making 18% of the runs and the ambulance service 82%.

PATIENT SERVICE: PUBLIC OR PRIVATE HOSPITALS

While some progress was being made in ambulance service, the patient, irrespective of the illness or injury, great or small, was being taken to the nearest hospital or to the hospital of his choice. No valid medical reasons governed these decisions. The surgeons on the medical society EMS committees were only too aware of the delays encountered in "cranking up the operating room" at night in most of the local hospitals to perform emergency surgery. Such delays coupled with inadequate x-ray and laboratory facilities and other instances when patients had been improperly handled suggested the need to categorize the hospital's ability to provide emergency health services and concentrate emergency care in appropriate institutions.

Transfer of Patients

Finances were another problem. The private hospitals in the city and county were delighted to be handed any well-heeled emergency patient, but when it turned out that the victim who had been dumped on their doorstep had no resources to compensate the staff and the hospital for the time and efforts extended in his care, they sought to transfer him by whatever means possible to the city or county hospitals.

The administrators of county hospitals were faced with declining patient populations, and were concerned that the acutely ill and injured patients should be taken to any private hospital in the first place. To encourage the private hospitals to get out of the emergency business, it was decided that private hospitals would have to pay for interhospital ambulance transfer. This decision resulted in a number of unfortunate events.

A robber and his intended victim, a grocer, exchanged shots. Both were taken to the same private hospital where the grocer was received, and care for his abdominal wound was started. The administrator of the hospital did not consider the robber of proper status for their institution despite his equal abdominal wounds, and they requested authority to transfer him to the county hospital. By authority to transfer is meant that the county would pay the ambulance charge. The county hospital administrator was not feeling too charitable on that day, and he told them that he would not pay for an ambulance, and if they wanted to transfer the robber they could do it at their own expense. Unbeknown to the county administrator, however, the private hospital had received authority shortly before this incident to transfer an auto-accident dead-on-arrival victim to the county hospital for autopsy by the coroner. The solution was immediately obvious to the private hospital. The wounded robber was placed in the ambulance with the dead accident victim and both were transported to the county hospital. Cries of anguish were heard in the press.

In another event a girl who had been stabbed multiple times in an attempted rape episode was taken to a local hospital. The night nursing supervisor was unfortunately in the emergency department and, being endowed with aged puritantic feelings, heard the word rape and screamed that the criminal girl should have been taken to the county hospital. She waved away all those who would unload the young woman and shooed off the ambulance. When the vehicle arrived at the county hospital, the girl was desparately ill from bilateral hemopneumothoraces and barely alive. A local newspaper sold a good many editions on their reporting of this unfortunate episode.

CATEGORIZATION OF HOSPITALS

At this point a set of guidelines for categorization of emergency facilities fell into the hands of the Emergency Medical Services Committee. These guidelines. as was learned later, were from a preliminary report that was never supposed to be released and had come out of the Committee on Trauma of the American College of Surgeons. How we ever got those guidelines has always been something of a mystery, but for those who have not had the opportunity to read this document let it be said that they were very stringent at the very least. A top-grade institution had to have immediately available cardiopulmonary bypass in addition to all the laboratory, operating-room, and other sophisticated ancillary services. The other guidelines for emergency facilities were almost equally rigid, so that in the metropolitan area, there were no hospitals that complied with category III, much less I, or II, guidelines.

A state of shock overtook the Metropolitan Hospital Association. A survey of the capabilities of the local hospitals was begun, and over half the hospitals had been evaluated before the remainder refused to cooperate. At the same time, physicians became increasingly concerned about what category might be ascribed to their primary institution.

Then the guidelines of EMS were provided by the American Medical Association.[5] To the already sensitized hospital administrators and their medical staffs, these guidelines loomed almost as threatening as those from the Ad Hoc Committee of the Committee on Trauma of the American College of Surgeons. But now the Metropolitan Hospital Association had recovered its usual obstructive functions and announced to any and all who would listen that they were working upon a system of categorization that would answer both the needs of the medical profession and yet allow for broader participation by its member hospitals. The hospital association had stumbled upon the categorization criteria used in San Diego, California.[14] Here were guidelines that most of its member hospitals could happily espouse, for basically what had been done was to remove the top two categories from the guidelines proposed from the AMA commission. Another committee of the Metropolitan Hospital Association was appointed, and multiple meetings again were held. This committee used a system similar to San Diego's provided criteria to categorize their hospitals.[4] A letter was sent with these criteria to all the member hospitals; it said, "Would you kindly survey your emergency medical facilities and write us a letter and tell us how you stand. Now we must warn you that there is a legal implication to this so be careful." This latter phrase scared the bejeepers out of most administrators, so nothing happened.

Then, as if to compound the difficulties, a few of the ambulances provided by the state and USDOT used their radios to communicate with receiving hospitals on the hospital radio network. Immediately the Metropolitan Hospital Association made it clear that their network was hospital disaster administrative and not to be used by ambulance personnel.

RESULTS

The results of 4 years of work by the joint Emergency Medical Services Committee could be summarized as follows:

1. An ambulance ordinance has been enacted in the city and county that defined the training and equipment of the various providers of ambulance services, but these ordinances had been largely ignored. Supervision in the county area of the ambulance providers was so spotty that, even though they were required to carry a minimum list of equipment, more than once it was considered very likely that the provider was sending one fully equipped ambulance in to be inspected, then taking the same equipment off that ambulance, and sending the next in for its annual inspection.
2. A training program had been provided for ambulance technicians, but because of the poor pay scale, the turnover of personnel was so rapid that it was almost impossible to keep trained ambulance technicians working.
3. The City of St. Louis ambulance service, as a transport mechanism for the acutely ill and injured, had been partially renovated but frequently was involved in fighting the police department to see who had the job of carrying the patient. The caliber of the men under the Emergency Employment Act was not too high, and moreover it was difficult for them to assimilate the training.
4. The Metropolitan Hospital Association had developed and implemented a communication network, but this network was not to be sullied by the use of ambulance personnel. Moreover most of the hospital receivers were installed in the administrator's office or in that of the telephone switchboard, so communication between the ambulance personnel and a physician in the emergency department of the receiving hospital was impossible.
5. The Metropolitan Hospital Association having decided to categorize its members had chosen inadequate categorization guidelines. Even these guidelines had been ignored by the members of the hospital association of the metropolitan area.

CITIZENS COMMITTEE

It was now realized that the time-honored citizens committee was the necessary route to follow. The membership of this committee was to be composed of anybody who seemed to have an interest in providing or receiving emergency medical service and care. Such a committee was formed and began to hold meetings once a month with its activities duly reported in the local press. This citizens committee, however, had no operating funds, and the secretarial service came from one of the medical societies, and the auditorium was provided by Washington University Medical School. A good executive secretary and staff were needed to develop surveys, training programs, and coordinated activities.

REGIONAL MEDICAL PROGRAMS

Then the Regional Medical Programs announced they would make part of $15 million available in five areas that could show some promise of developing an EMS system. The chairmen of the Emergency Medical Services Committee worked for long hours with staff personnel of the Bi-State Regional Medical Program and a grant application for $1.3 million was forwarded to Washington, D.C., in record time. The sites for funding were narrowed to eight, and a site visit was held in the St. Louis area.

As was commented upon later, that site visit truly reflected why a cohesive program had never developed. One local representative of government or hospital or ambulance service after another dutifully explained to the site team that they were wholly in accord with the concept of a unified approach, but in no way could such coordination change how they operated.

St. Louis was not chosen for funding of an EMS system, but as one of the site visitors noted afterward, the problems were so deep and reflected so many divergent views that consideration was given to funding the St. Louis area because it was felt that, if a system could be developed in this community, it could be developed with great ease anywhere else in the United States.

Although the St. Louis community did not get the $1.3 million, it did get $200,000 for planning and training.

Board of Directors

At this point the local governmental authorities decided that a board of directors was needed to oversee the expenditures of these funds, and a nonprofit corporation, Metropolitan Emergency Dispatch (MED) Inc., was established as an implementing agency. Persons to represent the government as well as the citizens were appointed. Expecting the Regional Medical Programs money, a search committee was appointed to look for an executive director for this new agency, but then the bolt of lightning struck from Washington. The $200,000 that had been allocated could not be spent; Regional Medical Programs were to be phased out. Having been cast into a financial limbo by the announcement that the program might be terminated, the political appointees felt that any activities were fruitless, and the best thing to do was to stop all efforts and forget about the whole thing. The citizens' appointees considered, on the other hand, that nobody has really stated that the money would never be allocated and that as long as there was any hope it would be well to be about their business and continue to look for an executive secretary.

The vacillations of Congress in terms of funding of Regional Medical Programs were equally reflected in the vacillations of the board of directors of MED Inc., and many a heated discussion ensued. In January 1973, when it became known that Regional Medical Programs would be funded for at least the next 6 months and that at least part of the $200,000 promised to MED Inc. would be forthcoming, it was decided to hire a permanent executive secretary. Finally, 5 years after our initial efforts had begun, the local area had one person who was an expert in the field and who had no commitments except that of developing a system of emergency medical care. This expert prompted a number of resignations from the board of MED Inc. (the recalcitrant directors), and new appointments were made; finally a board was developed with a true commitment to develop emergency medical services.

Training Programs

The training programs that had been produced by local physicians were inadequate to take care of the many people who might have something to do with the delivery of care on ambulances, and so a series of instructors lessons were begun. Already 500 potential ambulance technicians from all sources in the city and county have signed up for the program, and there will be 30 training programs of 81 hours covering these 500 men.

Hospital Categories

The hospital association pushed its members to accept the lax categorization standards, and suddenly 22 of 24 hospitals in the area found they were a number 1 facility. This kind of information was, to say the least, useless. To get around the problem of categorization of the hospitals, it was unofficially decided that those hospitals that had 24-hour operating-room coverage would be called trauma centers. The acutely ill and very severely injured would be taken to these designated (university and municipal) hospitals. Patients would be transported to other hospitals only when the patient demanded this service. It is hoped that this solution will be satisfactory to both the hospital association and to the general public.

RESEARCH TRAUMA CENTERS

True research trauma centers need to be developed in the university and municipal hospitals in the City of St. Louis. Possibly three other hospitals in the outlying areas should be developing such facilities. It is hoped that in the future helicopter transfer will be arranged so that people 100 or more miles from the City of St. Louis can be transferred to the metropolitan trauma centers. The government of the City of St. Louis made money available for more ambulances, and two are to have telemetry to manage cardiacs during transport. In St. Louis County the government belatedly realized that it was falling behind the city government, and they too stated their dedication to the development of an emergency medical care system with high standards. Some of these latter brave decisions were encouraged by the passage of an ambulance law by the State of Missouri that requires at least 44 hours of training (with the assumption that it would be raised to 81 hours within a year or 2) and requires ambulances to meet the standards promulgated by the National Academy of Sciences.[1]

911 SERVICE

The concept of the universal telephone number, 911, was studied soon after the formation of the Emergency Medical Services Committee.[2] In the City of St. Louis this system could easily be implemented, since there is one government with one police, fire, and ambulance service. But many of the telephone exchanges cover not only the city but also contiguous county communities. In some areas of the county the police and fire districts are not identical, and the ambulance areas also frequently overlap. A proposal has been made to implement an automated 911 system with as many as 40 dispatch centers. With this system, 911 could be dialed in the entire area, but the call would be routed automatically to the appropriate dispatch center for that call. This system is under study but costs would be high.

The boundaries of police, fire, and ambulance services also need to be revised so that they coincide. Some kind of overall coordination will also be necessary to know where all the ambulances are located to provide backup coverage when an ambulance is in service.

254

CONCLUSION

And so, as it was said in the beginning of this chapter, the odds are much better for your return to health or even your survival in the St. Louis metropolitan area now than was true several years ago. Much remains to be done but again let it be emphasized that many of the problems that were encountered could have been avoided had a good citizens committee been started early in the program design. This committee must clearly involve the mayors and other governmental authorities, so that it cannot be claimed later that the plan was not of their doing. Also this committee must have a paid executive secretary and staff who have no other jobs. This approach implies some funding source, and while start-up money may be available from the federal government,[9] in the long-run the money must come from the local government for the programs to continue. At the same time, if local officials put in their money it can be expected that they will insure the plan's success. We had been advised that this approach was the way to go but chose instead what was believed to be a shortcut, *e.g.*, design the system, then force the providers to accept it. This idea was no shortcut, but rather a quagmire. So while no one can point as yet to the St. Louis experience to illustrate what a good EMS system should be, the errors can be pointed out so that others may avoid similar mistakes in developing their own programs.

REFERENCES

[1] Ambulance design criteria, National Highway Safety Program, Washington, U.S. Department of Transportation, 1970

[2] Border KR, Huston JS: 911, a study of the single emergency telephone number. Philadelphia, Franklin Institute Research Laboratories, 1970

[3] Boyd DR: Statewide emergency medical care. J Trauma 13:275, 1973

[4] Categories of hospital emergency services in the St. Louis metropolitan area. St. Louis, Hospital Association of Metropolitan St. Louis, 1972

[5] Categorization of hospital emergency capabilities. Conference of the American Medical Association Commission on Emergency Medical Services, Chicago, 1971

[6] Committee on Trauma, American College of Surgeons: Essential equipment for ambulances. Bull Am Coll Surg, 155 (7), 1970

[7] Developing emergency medical services; guidelines for community councils. Chicago, Commission on Emergency Medical Services, American Medical Association, 1972

[8] Emergency care and transportation of the sick and injured. Committee on Injuries, American Academy of Orthopedic Surgeons, 1971

⁹ Emergency Medical Services Act of 1973. Public Law 93–154, Washington, 93rd Congress of the United States, 1973

¹⁰ Emergency medical services communications systems. Publication (HSM) 83–2003 Washington, U.S. Department of Health, Education, and Welfare, 1972

¹¹ Haeck WT: An emergency medical services system that works. J Am Hosp Assoc 47:139–142, 1973

¹² Hampton OP, Jr.: The systematic approach to EMS. Bull Am Coll Surg 53:231–233, 1968

¹³ Klippel AP: Emergency medical services, practice of surgery, vol. II. St. Louis, C.V. Mosby, 1974

¹⁴ Murray SP: San Diego plan for emergency services. Am J Nurs 72:1615–1619, 1972

¹⁵ National Highway Traffic Safety Administration. Basic training program for emergency medical technicians—ambulance. Instructor's lesson plans. Washington, U.S. Department of Transportation, 1971

Sam Landrum
Dan J. Scott, Jr.

21

Emergency Medical Service Councils

Until recently, components of EMS systems were developed in many communities and a few wide areas. Usually, these components were specialized components of variable quality related to a limited part of an overall EMS system, the emphasis being on equipment, on advanced training of EMTs, or on communication.

Development of systems with excellence in all components is rare. This rarity is probably related to the fact that many motivated, enthusiastic persons, agencies, or institutions have endeavored to meet the EMS needs on the basis of their own individual viewpoints or principal interests. Thus, hospitals provided emergency rooms; professional organizations have conducted training by those few of their number who were interested in providing EMS. Biomedical engineers and manufacturers brought out highly technical and useful equipment for communication and treatment, courses for EMTs were offered, and planners produced volumes to be reviewed and commented upon by others at multiple conferences and by countless editors. However, those responsible for one facet were not aware or very inquisitive of what was being done by those interested in another facet. Hence, the quality and availability of EMS have been excellent in a few areas, spotty in other areas, and nonexistent in others.

Councils of EMS at the local level will determine the actual services that a citizen can expect. These councils will be charged with the responsibility of delivering health care to the people, who must be educated that they need this care and must be willing to pay for it. The geographic size that the area serves will be influenced by the economics and population density of the area. Obviously, a small area cannot afford the expense of vehicles, communication equipment, salaries, and training of personnel. The council will, of necessity, have to cut across county and state boundaries to render the most effective EMS without their being prohibitively expensive and with the cooperation of all involved segments.

COMPONENTS OF EMS COUNCILS

Initially, it was felt that councils would best be free-standing with representation from all groups responsible for the delivery of health care. This type of council would have no authority, however, and probably no lasting role in the area it would serve. The Emergency Medical Service Systems Act of 1973 (Public Law 93-154) stipulates that funds to local areas be processed with comprehensive health planning A and B agencies. A local authority under the present law would be in conflict with comprehensive health planning agencies. It appears that the federal agencies are to plan all emergency medical service in their area. Implementation of these plans will still depend on the delivery of a patient to a hospital. As the safe delivery of this patient in the best possible condition with the best possible care is the ultimate goal, the suppliers of the various components should find a way to work together. These basic components are medical self-help, communications, EMTs, emergency vehicles, emergency department, and hospital physicians, nurses, and other personnel.

FUNDING SOURCES

It appears very likely that the federal government will assume control of all prehospital EMS. Under these circumstances it would be prudent to combine all the government monies for EMS under one director. If comprehensive health planning agencies are to continue under the direction of the Department of Health, Education, and Welfare, it would seem logical that they would furnish the necessary housing and secretarial help to the council. Councils set up under separate autonomous authority would, of necessity, look to other sources for grants, that is, state and local government and private monies.

RESPONSIBILITIES

The major responsibilities of the EMS council are to coordinate EMS activities in its area to prevent duplication, to help correct and identify any shortcomings in any components of its system, and to produce a system that can care for the individual but expand to meet the mass casualty situation. The council would also coordinate its activities with adjoining areas. Only by coordination will the delivery of EMS be orderly, efficient, and without prohibitive expenses. The expected results would be

1. Reduction of operational expenses for smaller areas that could not afford their own ambulances and equipment
2. Standardization of EMT training
3. Possible establishment of emergency care centers to make the best use of personnel
4. Expansion of EMS to meet disaster situations
5. To have one responsible body to make decisions and be answerable to the public
6. Evaluation of cost effectiveness in the community
7. To plan for improvement and projected needs
8. To direct lay education through schools and with the help of service clubs

COMPONENTS CONTROLLED BY THE COUNCIL

Prior to the passage of the Emergency Medical Services Act of 1973, it was felt that the council should have the authority to implement an EMS system and be able by law to collect grants and fees and to own and lease property. Since the passage of the 1973 law, it appears that the council will be an advisory body to the government agency designated responsible for EMS in the area it encompasses.

It should not be the function of the council to control but to offer expert advice and to ascertain that the best possible EMS is being rendered to citizens and their community. The councils, to be effective, must be completely altruistic. Their control should be through the highest ideals espoused by the members of the organization represented on the council.

In some areas the councils may function as independent authorities, however; if they have no power to implement their proposals the councils would be meaningless. The representatives should have authority from the highest possible source in their local government. It would be well if local governments would cooperate and set aside the money needed to implement their councils' decisions. In those areas in which this provision is impossible, local authorities established by state or federal legislature may be necessary. Withholding state and federal funds would be necessary on some occasions to coax some areas into compliance. The EMS areas that strive without prodding and with their own resources would therefore be less dependent on outside sources in meeting their needs as they see fit.

The representatives appointed to a council should be appointed by job or organization rather than by name, as organizations live longer than people as a rule. Each member should have equal voice. As a representative of a larger group, information from the council will be widely disseminated and collected, as seen in Figure 21.1. The spin-off to and from the involved organization is vital to the function of this council.

Each state is divided into developmental districts, and within these districts are comprehensive health planning B agencies with a professional staff capable of surveying the needs of an area. The development district director should know the members of local government who should be represented. The heads of the development districts and comprehensive health planning agencies should be represented on the council and should be expected to furnish needed support to implement the council's determinations.

An autonomous council should have the authority to collect money and disperse grants and fees; to own and lease property, such as ambulances, communication equipment, and teaching aids; and to enforce their decisions through the representative of government on the council. Such a council by having representatives of government, business, and allied medical personnel will provide its own checks and balances to prevent the formation of an autocratic monster.

MEMBERSHIP AND REPRESENTATION

The council members should be from the medical community, government, and business to keep it well balanced and attuned to the needs of the community it serves. A consumer who has utilized the services

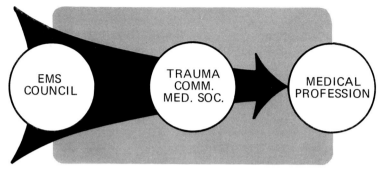

Figure 21.1
The collection and dissemination of information by the EMS council.

should also be included to keep the council in a level and pragmatic position (Fig. 21.2).

A State council should be kept small and composed of representatives of the state medical association, nurses association, hospital association, ambulance operators, and officials of government.

On the national council, there should be representation from all national organizations concerned with EMS, such as the AMA, the American Academy of Orthopedic Surgeons, the American College of Surgeons, the American Hospital Association, the American Nurses Association, civil defense, and the Red Cross.

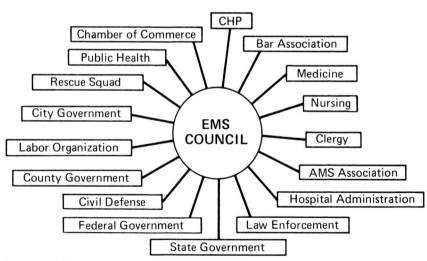

Figure 21.2
Representation on the EMS council.

This council should establish policies that the state can implement as they see fit and can afford. The states should not set conflicting ideals or policies. Through this council, all the components of an effective national EMS can be coordinated and guidance furnished to all levels. This council should be expected to furnish the goals that the states strive to meet through local councils.

COMMUNITY SUPPORT

As the public becomes more aware of its health needs, they will demand more and better care in all areas of services. In some areas this will take much longer because of economics and geography. In all areas an effective council with broad representation will engender a broad base of community support. Representatives of business, clergy, educators, and the legal profession will serve to keep the council oriented to the public needs.

SUBCOMMITTEES

As the council matures and goals are met, certain subcommittees may need to be phased out. New needs may also arise, which would require the information of new subcommittees.

Subdivision of the council into subcommittees concerned with various facets of EMS will save the time of the whole council and lend more expertise to problem solution. The various committees and their representatives are as follows:

1. Initial emergency care (medical self-help): comprehensive health planners, clergy, Red Cross, schools, and public health
2. Communication: civil defense, telephone company, hospital administration, fire department, highway patrol, state, comprehensive health planners, Red Cross, EMTs, ambulance association, nurses, and medical society
3. Vehicle: ambulance association, EMTs, medical society, and police and fire department
4. Emergency department:˙ hospital administration, ambulance services, EMTs, nurses, and physicians
5. Disaster medicine: civil defense, law enforcement, ambulance association, Red Cross, hospital administration, physicians, public health, and local government
6. Disaster coordination: civil defense, city government, county government, school, clergy, utilities, telephone, fire, law enforcement, public health, hospital administration, and business

LOCATION OF THE COUNCIL

After the passage of the Emergency Medical Services Systems Act of 1973, the national EMS council will be under the supervision of the Department of Health, Education, and Welfare. This supervision does not preclude the formation of a free-standing EMS council with representatives of prestigious organizations such as the American College of Surgeons, the American Academy of Orthopedic Surgeons, the AMA, the American Hospital Association, the American Nurses Association, and the Red Cross, to list only a few. This council can be most effective in providing expert advice that cannot be purchased. In the education of the EMTs, nurses, and physicians and in setting standards of excellence for the hospital and health personnel, this body would be of the greatest importance.

At a state level, the council should be a separate agency of the governor's office or come under the Department of Public Health or Highway Safety. The organization and operational complexity of a state EMS system necessitate the creation of an EMS planning and coordination unit. As the unit functions in the realm of public health, an effective public health department probably should be given first consideration.

Local councils with free-standing authority, should have the support and funds available to provide their own housing and staff. If the council is to work closely with the comprehensive health-planning agency or area development district, then either of these agencies could be expected to furnish staff support. Much now depends on interpretation of the Emergency Medical Services Systems Act of 1973. It should be noted at this point that prehospital EMS could function very well without support of the medical community. Since we are interested in the patient's care after his delivery to the emergency department, continued high motivation of the physician, nurse, and paramedical personnel is a must and should be considered in any planning.

RESPONSIBILITIES ACCORDING
TO GOVERNMENT LEVEL

The responsibilities of the local council have been discussed earlier; those of the state or national EMS councils depend on the passage of effective legislature at both levels. No implementation can succeed in the long run if there are no laws stating who is responsible for implementing a council's deliberations, no matter how wise they are.

The state council will not be effective if it is not privy to information and facts. A plan to coordinate immediate and long-range goals with comprehensive health planning A agencies should be developed after the state needs have been surveyed. Medical self-help programs should be developed and additional legislature planned as indicated. Communication needs should be considered and coordinated in the department. The emergency vehicle can be regulated according to type, equipment, and inspection. The emergency vehicle operators and EMTs should be required to meet certain regulations, and the EMTs should be encouraged to join the National Registry. These regulations, of course, include licensing of the vehicles, the operators, and the EMTs.

Penalties and appeals should be considered on individual merit. The state EMS council should consider a uniform state categorization of emergency departments in cooperation with the state hospital association and medical association. Provisions for periodic reevaluation of various components should be mandatory, and interstate cooperation should be stressed. Each state EMS council should be prepared to help the local EMS councils find the ways and means to make themselves effective councils for the public good.

The goal of a national council should be to standardize EMS throughout the country at the highest possible level. The council and the EMS system serve to coordinate all of the various programs that have been instituted in various governmental departments. Through this service a national trauma registry should be formed that allows us to know how effective EMS is in reducing mortality and morbidity and, thus, how to increase its effectiveness. It is hoped that, through this coordination, wasteful expenditure of funds can be avoided and that conflicts of interest and petty jealousy can be avoided. This national council should be expected to set the goals that state and local councils strive to meet. The council should continue throughout its function to coordinate all EMS components in this country and furnish guidance at all component levels.

Francis C. Jackson

22

Airport Emergency and Disaster Preparedness Planning

Described as the pulse of their cities' heartbeat, airports and the air-carrier operations have become the tenth largest industry in the nation. In addition, major airports serve their cities well; San Francisco's International Airport generates over $13 billion for the city each year. Prior to the energy crisis in the winter of 1973–1974, federal authorities were predicting that the 10% annual growth rate of domestic air travel would continue into the 1980s when an incredible 500,000,000 travelers would be expected to take to the airways each year.[21]

The major airport is a complex organization to control and operate. Usually owned and operated by a local government or a public authority, it provides a variety of services for its commercial tenants, the air carriers. All must function under a wide range of federal laws, rules, and regulations. Needless to say, any emergency or major catastrophe that occurs in such a setting could result in chaos, and indeed it frequently does. Airports have been called, not improperly, "thresholds of disaster."[15]

RULES, REGULATIONS, AND REGULATORS

The first federal agency given the responsibility by the Congress to control and regulate commercial air travel was the Civil Aeronautics Board (CAB) founded in 1938. It was (and is) mainly responsible for insuring that the airlines offer safe services and that reasonable rates are charged. The CAB also assigns intercity air routes and to a large extent successfully insures and even controls competition.

In 1958 the Federal Aviation Administration (FAA) was created with power to supervise and certify aircraft and aircraft manufacturing and engineering, aircraft repair and maintenance facilities, aircraft operation, pilot certificates, and pilot training schools. The agency also controls the efficient use of and safety within the air space used by civil aircraft.

Public Law 91–258, the Airport and Airway Development Act passed by the Congress in 1970, authorized the FAA, for the first time, to issue airport operating certificates for those airports serving air carriers certified by the CAB and to establish minimum safety standards for their operation. Since May 1973, no certified air carrier is permitted to use an airfield that does not hold such an operating certificate.

Section 139.55 of the FAA Regulations that govern airport certification requires airport operators of air-carrier airports to maintain an emergency plan that is sufficiently detailed to provide adequate guidance in response to all emergencies. In addition, the operator "must show that before applying, he has coordinated the emergency plan with law enforcement, fire fighting, and rescue agencies, medical resources, the principal tenants at the airport, and other interested persons.[24]"

Provisions in the regulation specifically call for the emergency plan to carry detailed instructions for aircraft incidents and accidents, bomb threats, structural fires, natural disasters, sabotage, radiologic incidents (including a nuclear attack), emergency medical services, crowd control, removal of disabled aircraft, emergency alarm systems, mutual assistance agreements with local safety and security agencies, and emergency functions of the airport and control tower. The regulation somewhat pointedly urges that all airport personnel, with emergency roles, must be "familiar with their assignments and properly trained." Unfortunately, the greatest weakness in these regulations is a failure to require air-carrier airports to rehearse such emergency and disaster plans on a regular basis.

When being certified, the airport operator must also submit an "Operations Manual" for approval by the FAA; the manual must indicate compliance with all provisions of Section 139.55. The Aeromedical Services Division of the FAA reviews the medical services portion of the airport manual of operations and is available for assistance and guidance in its development or revision. The document finally becomes a part of the operating certificate, which is available for public inspection as well as subject to administrative and judicial sanctions if violated. The FAA periodically issues circulars to provide additional help in these matters.[4,5,11]

The most recent federal organization to evolve in the evolution of regulated public transportation and the first to be primarily responsible for safety is the National Transportation Safety Board (NTSB) created in 1967. One of the agency's roles is to determine the cause(s) of all transportation accidents and to recommend corrective actions. The board's headquarters is in Washington, D.C., where it maintains a ten-man "go-team" of technicians to investigate all air-carrier accidents with fatalities. The team assumes complete charge of a crash area. Even the wreckage becomes the property of the NTSB until it is released.[9]

Technical assistance relating to injury and fatality analysis in such onsite investigations is furnished to the "go-team" by a "human factors group" usually chaired by a member of the Human Factors Branch of the NTSB. Other members include representatives from the Office of Aviation Medicine (FAA), the Civil Aeromedical Institute (FAA-CAMI), the Airline Pilots Association (ALPA), and the involved airline. The pharmacology-biochemical laboratories of the FAA-CAMI and the Armed Forces Institute of Pathology provide the necessary blood chemistry and histologic analyses on the remains of air crews and passengers. The drug and alcohol contents in the blood of pilots and the level of carboxyhemoglobin in the tissues of the dead aid in the search for human causes of accidents and the mechanisms of lethal injury. These investigators also determine whether such accidents are survivable or nonsurvivable by noting the breakup characteristics of the aircraft.[9,10,25,26,27,28,29]

The onsite investigations are also followed by public hearings in which all evidence of the accident is presented in sworn testimony. Physicians and others concerned with emergency planning for aircraft disasters should attend one of these hearings.

It is unfortunate that when all the evidence relating to given aircraft catastrophies is presented and reviewed by competent NTSB experts, their recommendations to improve the safety of aircraft operations are not mandatory upon the FAA. Corrections in dangerous structural features of airliners or the required addition of new safety devices are occasionally delayed before adoption by this agency.

DAILY EMERGENCY SERVICES AND MEDICAL FACILITIES

Even though all airline airports are publicly operated and have the responsibility of providing services, it is the passenger volume of air-carrier operations that governs the size, staffing, and services rendered by the emergency unit.

The FAA classifies airfields into large, medium, and small airports depending on the percentage of all U.S. passengers enplaned using that particular field in a given year. To be rated as a large airport in 1974, the field must serve over 1% of all airline passengers that year; a medium-sized field must serve 0.25–0.99%, and a small airport services between 0.05 and 0.24% of nation-wide air travelers.

The medical and emergency services at 21 geographically selected airports in all three classes were surveyed by two federal agencies in 1972.[19] Although the report is unpublished and its results must be reviewed with caution, they nevertheless support the observations and impressions of this author and others, namely, that airports prior to the new FAA certification requirements, for the most part, gave little priority to their EMS system and disaster planning.[13,23,31] This finding has been substantiated more recently at a conference conducted by the National Health Resources Advisory Committee of the Office of Preparedness in the General Services Administration.[24]

The unpublished report noted that of seven large airfields, only four supplied emergency medical aid to the public. Of 13 medium and small air-carrier airfields, only six had first-aid facilities. The airport authority is responsible for insuring the availability of these services; yet the units are generally only attended by nurses and first-aid personnel. Few airports provide services through a medical concessionaire. The airlines occasionally have medical offices whose principal activities are related more to aviation medicine than to caring for the needs of travelers. However, the major deficiency at most of the world's airport health facilities is the unavailability of physicians.[18]

Of course the demands for medical care at airports provide few challenges for physicians. Poor recruitment is related to the low volume and the infrequency of challenging problems among transients and airport employees. Even though only the fit tend to travel, both the

FAA and the air carriers restrict certain ill and chronically disabled persons from boarding commercial aircraft, a practice that has encouraged the development of air charter ambulance services. In addition to these restrictions, other FAA regulations require manufacturers to design aircraft and the airlines to train their crews so that all able passengers can be evacuated within 90 sec during an emergency. A passenger's obvious inability to carry out this feat becomes a strong deterrent to the airline's issuance of a ticket. The pilot has the final say, however.

Nevertheless, major airports can have relatively busy health facilities. O'Hare International Airport (the world's largest operator with an average of 97,000 air travelers daily) is without a physician; yet over 10,000 persons were treated in 1969 at its two aid stations; two-thirds of these were travelers and the rest employees. Five percent of those treated were transferred to hospitals or doctors' offices.[14]

Although airport operators studiously avoid any suggestion that they must engage in medical practice for the convenience of the public, they are nonetheless required to insure the availability of such services.[5]

Agreements, therefore, must exist between airport operators and airline tenants, medical concessionaires operating clinics, local hospitals, and ambulance services to meet most emergency needs. Many clinics on airport grounds are now successfully operated under national standards for such services.[4,12,17,18,20]

Important in the support of airport aid stations are ambulance services and community hospitals. For example, O'Hare Airport must transport by ambulance at least 40% of those requiring additional medical care. However, only 4 of the 21 fields in the survey reported that these vehicles were stationed on the grounds; three had helicopters available for such transfers. Ambulances on call were generally 10 min driving time away, while hospitals averaged 7 miles in distance from all fields. Irrespective of the circumstances, the time elapse between the call by the airport aid station to the ambulance dispatcher and the arrival of a casualty or acutely ill person at the hospital could easily exceed 30 min or more, depending on traffic conditions. This rate would suggest that more medical capability including life-support services should be required at all major airfields.

The J. F. Kennedy International Airport, on the other hand, has an unusually large medical facility that has grown since 1950. This medical office is operated under a concession and employs a staff of over 80 with 17 physicians, 1 on whom is always on duty. It also maintains a 20-bed treatment ward and mans an innovative mobile inflatable treatment unit (MITU) used by the Port Authority following disasters.[1,2]

AIRCRAFT DISASTERS IN THE UNITED STATES

Information on commercial aircraft accidents in this country is not easily obtained. While the Federal Aviation Administration (CAB) conducted investigations prior to 1967, the establishment of NTSB in that year has resulted in more comprehensive and generally more objective studies of causes and prevention. Such official reports are now available through the National Technical Information Service. However, epidemiologic information is still not published regularly.[6]

Aircraft accident data are studied by the NTSB according to services provided by six different classes of operators under two major groups: the commercial route carriers and the supplemental operators (*i.e.,* charter and military).[6] The largest volume of air traffic and the group of most concern in accident investigations are the scheduled domestic and international passenger services.

Between 1966 and 1972 an annual average of 55 aircraft accidents were investigated by the NTSB. The number of accidents with fatal injuries to passengers or crew approximated 12 per year during the same period (Table 22.1).

Table 22.1. Aircraft Fatalities in the United States, 1966–1972

	Accidents	Total	Average per year
Air Carrier Aviation	Total accidents	332	55
	—with fatalities	69 (21%)	12
	—with fatalities at airports	24 (7%)	4
	Total fatalities	1,587*	264
	—passengers	1,247 (79%)	208
	—crew	189 (12%)	32
	—others	151 (9%)	25
General Aviation	Total accidents	30,923†	5,154
	—with fatalities	3,818 (12%)	636
	—with fatalities at airports	366 (1%)	61

* Deaths as a result of aircraft accidents at the airport or in suburban areas near the airport.

† Classification of damage criteria for general aviation accidents was changed in 1967, resulting in an overall drop of 20% in the total number reported. However, the data on fatalities was unaffected.

General aviation in that time accounted for over 5,000 accidents per year, with more than 600 annual deaths.

While the airline industry was increasing its hours of operation, its number of departures, and air-carrier miles flown through 1969, the accident rate was actually decreasing for both total accidents and fatal accidents during the same 6-year period (Fig. 22.1). By that same year the accident rate was 0.023 and the fatality rate 0.003 per million aircraft miles flown.

A report by the NTSB published in 1971 carefully analyzed the 63 air-carrier accidents (ten with fatalities) that had occurred in 1969.[6] In the 63 accidents, the planes were either totally destroyed or sustained substantial damage in 35 instances. There were 158 fatalities, 71 serious injuries, and 3856 minor or no injuries to the passengers and crew.

It is of interest that the most commonly reported incident producing serious injuries (but no fatalities) is not takeoff or landing accident but air turbulence in flight. This type of misadventure to air travelers caused one-third of the injuries in 1969.

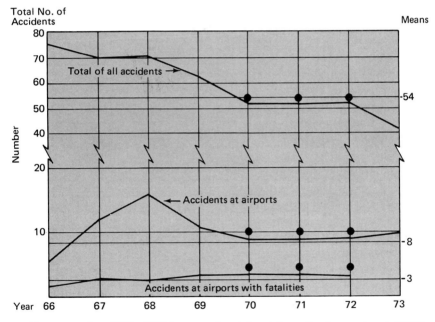

● Three years data, 1970 - 1972, is proportioned since information by year is unavailable

Figure 22.1
The number of air carrier accidents at U.S. airports has not been increasing. However, the appreciable number that does occur requires better planning and preparation than previously given.

AIRPORT DISASTERS

Approximately 20% of airline accidents occur at airfields, while an additional 40% of aircraft impact within 25 miles of these approach or takeoff operations. One-third of the commercial accidents on the airport grounds results in fatalities. While the total number of all aircraft accidents has shown a continuous decline since 1966, the airport incidents have exhibited little change, averaging about eight per year, with three producing some fatalities (Fig. 22.1).

In 140 consecutive commercial airline disasters occurring at airports in the 5-year period 1968–1972, 7600 passengers were at risk in 17 accidents. There were 115 deaths and 556 injuries, 30% of them serious. Four examples of these accidents will illustrate the problems they present to airport operators and disaster planners.

Crash 1

Late in 1965 a Boeing 727 landed hard and short of the runway of a medium-sized Western airport. One engine separated from the aircraft and the right main landing gear assembly punctured the fuselage, severing fuel lines and starting an immediate cabin fire. Since the impact forces were mild, the damaged and burning aircraft took almost 50 sec to come to a halt. Evacuation of passengers, already hampered by the fire and toxic gases was further delayed by failure of the main lighting system.[10] Among the 85 passengers, there were 43 deaths, despite the fact that all survived the initial impact. Those able to evacuate were principally young males seated near exits. Many of those with the fewest injuries had had occupational training in emergency and safety procedures, such as military or airline personnel and mining engineers. The principal mechanisms of the fatal injuries were chemical (hydrogen cyanide) and thermal damage to the respiratory tract, producing a choking laryngospasm. While over one-half of the dead received burns, only six of these were third degree. Seven passengers, seated forward of the fourth row, escaped with only vertebral fractures occurring at the time of the initial impact. All, except three survivors, evacuated themselves; the three were caught in the aft stairwell for almost 30 min before being rescued. Only nine survivors (10%) were essentially uninjured.[22,27]

In one official report of this catastrophe, problems common to most disasters were mentioned. These problems included alerting and coordinating the emergency response of 18 airport services, maintaining traffic and crowd control, and locating emergency equipment and other logistic support stored at the airfield.

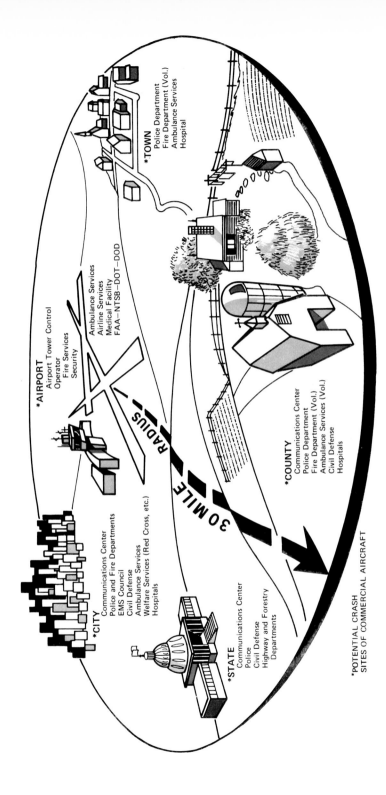

AIRPORT
Airport Tower Control
Operator
Fire Services
Security

Ambulance Services
Airline Services
Medical Facility
FAA–NTSB–DOT–DOD

*TOWN
Police Department
Fire Department (Vol.)
Ambulance Services
Hospital

*CITY
Communications Center
Police and Fire Departments
EMS Council
Civil Defense
Ambulance Services
Welfare Services (Red Cross, etc.)
Hospitals

*COUNTY
Communications Center
Police Department
Fire Department (Vol.)
Ambulance Services (Vol.)
Civil Defense
Hospitals

*STATE
Communications Center
Police
Civil Defense
Highway and Forestry
Departments

30 MILE RADIUS

*POTENTIAL CRASH
SITES OF COMMERCIAL AIRCRAFT

Figure 22.2
Aircraft on descent and take-off follow assigned routes relating to the runway compass headings, which, in the 30-mile area of tower control, extend as "air corridors" over many political subdivisions. Careful coordination of many agencies is necessary if disaster management is to be successful.

273

Crashes 2 and 3

During the year-end holidays and within 13 days of each other, two turboprop aircraft (Convair 580s) attempting landings in snowstorms, crashed short of the opposite ends of the same runway at an Eastern airport. These two accidents were studied in some depth by the NTSB and the U.S. Public Health Service. Interest in the latter agency was heightened by the similarity of the accidents and the intriguing question whether emergency services following the second crash were improved by lessons learned during the first.

Both aircraft were flying with zero visibility, on instruments, and were well below the designated altitudes. The airport did not have an Instrument Landing System (ILS). Its flight service station operated a simple directional range finder and only provided pilots with visibility and ceiling information. Visibility was 1 mile and the ceiling 400 ft at the time of the subject accidents. The first accident occurred in a remote mountain marsh and the second on a golf course, 1 and 5 miles short on the approach to the runway. Both lost a wing in trees then quickly overturned, and impacted on their cabin roofs. There was no appreciable fire in either instance.

A total of 75 passengers and crew in both aircraft were at risk, of whom 44 (59%) survived. All deaths occurring at the scenes were due to massive crush injuries to the head and thorax. These victims were located in the forward overturned cabins where the greatest impact forces occurred.[16]

This airport, because of its small size (13 daily commercial flights), had no disaster plan other than an alerting system, and its closest fire and ambulance services were 5 miles distant. The principal of two hospitals was 20 miles away. Local authorities provided little coordinating assistance to the many units and agencies arriving at the scene of the accidents. The responding ambulance companies were not under firm leadership and neither the civil defense director nor the state police assumed this responsibility at the disaster sites. A call for more assistance through the news media led to crowd convergence and looting. Authorities also failed to adhere to the coroner's regulations regarding the handling of the dead, and there was no coordination among ambulance services in the distribution of survivors. Rescue efforts were so poorly accomplished that the last survivors were not removed from the first accident until 5 hours after the crash. Although first-aid services were not provided at the scene before transportation to the hospitals, the hospitals were able to efficiently organize their staff operations, since the arrival of casualties was intermittent and widespaced after the initial alert. Nine survivors were operated upon under local anesthesia.

There were three seriously and permanently injured passengers, but all survived to leave the hospital.

Crash 4

In December 1972, the first "Jumbo Jet" accident in the United States with fatalities occurred in Florida. The plane had been diverted from the field because of difficulty in confirming that the nose wheel was in the locked-down position. The actual crash occurred when the air crew did not monitor flight instruments during the final 4 minutes before landing and failed to detect the craft's slow and progressive descent into the darkened Everglade marshes.

While the airport operators had a well-developed disaster plan, the distance of the crash site from the field placed the emergency assistance responsibilities, as well as the rescue and medical operations, in the hands of county authorities. However, the airport approach controller performed a major communications feat by coordinating many emergency agencies which had access to his tower radio frequencies and the general telephone system.

Most of the survivors were located in the vicinity of the cockpit area, mid-cabin service area, the overwing area and the empennage section. The fatal injuries occurred in the center of the crash path. Deaths resulted principally from crushing chest injuries.

Sixty-seven (38%) of the 176 passengers and crew were immediate survivors; a particularly large group considering the complete fragmentation of the aircraft. This large jet aircraft demonstrated its capability of absorbing many of the impact forces previously considered insurvivable.[3]

The problems encountered with this accident were unique to the difficult and marshy terrain, to the insufficient illumination for night rescue operations, to the incompatibility of radio frequencies, and to the lack of centralized control of rescue operations. The inability to triage and provide immediate treatment for the survivors at the scene was particularly discouraging to the several experienced physicians who went immediately to the scene. The fact that the county government did not have a disaster plan known to all other agencies was a particular deficiency.

Commendable in the rescue operations, however, was the efficient use of four helicopters by the U.S. Coast Guard, which provided air control over the site and some illumination ("nite sun"), as well as transporting rescue personnel, supplies, and 42% or 63% of all survivors to nearby hospitals.

ESTIMATING DEATHS AND INJURIES

Estimating the total number of casualties and the proportions among types of injuries occurring in aircraft accidents is theoretically helpful in planning for the organization of emergency medical operations, such as making personnel assignments and ordering equipment or supplies for storage. It could also permit the roles of each local hospital to be determined and permit the distribution of casualties among them (*i.e.*, if their emergency capabilities are classified).

It has correctly been pointed out that the number and severity of injuries is affected by many variables including such elements as the type of aircraft; the time and site of the accident; whether the aircraft disintegrated, exploded, or caught fire; the severity of deceleration effects; the personal behavior and physical arrangement of the passengers in the cabin; the discipline of the flight personnel; and the efficiency of the rescue operations.[30] Generally, these observations have been borne out in the medical and human factor studies conducted by the NTSB as well as in tests by aviation laboratories.

A common sequence for a serious injury is initiated when the individual is jack-knifed on the seat belt. The flaying arms and legs are traumatized on the sharp edges of the forward seat, while the head strikes the upright serving tray. Further, the unfortunate passenger may sustain fractures of the lower leg and be sufficiently stunned so as to be totally immobilized during the critical moments of evacuation or rescue, particularly if a fire begins to engulf the damaged cabin.

For disaster planners the most important preliminary information would be an estimate of the total numbers of survivors to be expected following those accidents limited to the airport grounds. The largest survivorship should occur in these instances and, therefore, the maximum numbers for disaster planning purposes. The second most important planning information to have available would be an estimate of the distribution of injuries among the survivors.

Bergot, who has developed an elaborate emergency organization for the airports serving Paris, recommended that the passenger capacity of the largest plane using the airport ("critical medical aircraft") be used in such determinations. After comprehensive studies of aircraft disasters within 9 km of these airports, he suggested that airport planning for casualty care should be based on the expectation that 40% of the passengers in the "critical medical aircraft" would survive the immediate crash.[7]

Since Bergot's estimates were based on experience with airliners operating before the wide-body jet aircraft were in common use, his predictions may be too low. The Jumbo Jet may absorb more forces of impact as evidenced by the Lockheed L-1011 accident described previously. This accident was considered nonsurvivable; yet 38% passengers and crew were alive at the scene. Nonetheless, any plan based upon services, supplies, and equipment for 40–50% of the passenger-carrying capacity of the largest plane using any field should be a sufficiently adequate planning base until better working information is available.

Knowledge of the expected frequency within a spectrum of injuries, as mentioned, could be more helpful. Unfortunately, the distribution of these injuries to the lower extremities, upper extremities, chest and abdomen, spine, face, and head does not form a recurring pattern. Concussion, burns, and smoke inhalation may complicate these skeletal injuries and seriously hamper the victim's efforts to evacuate himself. Trauma from seat belts or that occurring during the rescue efforts may be superimposed after the initial impact. If there is no fire, inhalation and respiratory difficulties are not encountered. Injuries also occur from detachment of seats (inadequate "tie down"), from missiles within the cabin, and with collapse of the fuselage airframe.[8]

Survival has also been related to age (the elderly and children fail to evacuate), sex (females are frequently unable to overcome the obstacle of evacuation), seating location (near exits), occupational experience (military discipline aids in emergencies), and selective capability of surviving with multiple injuries long enough to be hospitalized. Essentially all survivors arriving at a medical center live through their experience.

Bergot also made the following assumptions: 10% of survivors will have life-threatening injuries or complications requiring on-site care; 20% will be moderately injured and will require hospitalization; and 70% will have minor injuries requiring little or no treatment. For a Boeing 747, he estimates that there would be 15, 30, and 95 survivors, respectively, in each of these categories. His assumptions, while arbitrary, are, I believe, appropriate for planning purposes. Most air carriers request, and planners should be prepared to implement, the admission of most survivors to hospitals. Irrespective of the causes of air accidents, they are generally considered "man-made" until proven otherwise by an official investigation. All hospital records become important legal documents.

DEVELOPING AN AIRPORT DISASTER PLAN

Before attempting to develop or revise an existing medical annex to the airport disaster plan, the following steps should be taken: (1) a review of FAA regulations and emergency planning circulars; [4,5,11,24]

(2) a review of the National Health Resources Advisory Committee "Report on Airport/Community Emergency Medical Preparedness;"[21] (3) a review of the subject airport's existing general emergency plan (nonmedical portion); (4) a review of selected disaster plans of other airports (in the opinion of the author the best of eight plans reviewed for this report are those prepared at Dallas–Ft. Worth and Baltimore–Washington airports); (5) prepare an inventory of all emergency medical resources in the community; (6) request the assistance and support of the community's council on EMS in the community; (7) write a plan using the check list provided in Appendix A and circulate a draft of the document to all concerned, including outside consultants; (8) rehearse the final plan regularly, rewriting and improving it as experience dictates; and (9) study official reports of airport air-carrier accidents.

Probably the most important effort on the part of the airport's medical planner is to gain the respect, confidence, and support of the airport operator, the air carriers, the Airline Pilot's Association, governmental agencies (police and fire), community welfare services, and the health professional groups including the hospital council.

A major concern is reaching an agreement on disaster site command responsibilities, *i.e.*, at the scene and at a centralized emergency operations center. Well-meaning fire, police, and health authorities representing political subdivisions can create almost insurmountable problems when the accident occurs in one of their communities along the 30-mile approach to the major runways. The political groups and involved agencies of the various governmental authorities are identified in Figure 22.2. All must be involved in developing a workable area-wide plan for aircraft accidents.

The coordination of these elements is vital to the success of any plan. In particular, it is important that the authority and responsibility of the medical coordinator or disaster director be recognized at all levels within the command structure and wherever the accident has occurred. The peculiar complexities of airport disaster planning was recognized by the Federal Office of Preparedness, which held an important national conference on the subject in Chicago, Illinois, in the fall of 1973.

THE NATIONAL HEALTH RESOURCES ADVISORY COMMITTEE

The National Health Resources Advisory Committee is a major advisory group to the Office of Preparedness in the General Services Administration. In October 1973, the committee, which is concerned with a continuing review of all federal planning for emergency and disaster services, developed three major recommendations for improving airport and community emergency medical preparedness. With the aid of 60 experts from government, aviation, and medicine, the committee also reached a number of basic conclusions and made innumerable recommendations.[21]

The document reported that more comprehensive emergency planning for airport emergencies was necessary, that a systems approach was required, that the Federal government should take more action using public and private expertise, that airport plans should be more closely linked to those of their communities, that political jurisdictional problems should be resolved with mutual aid agreements (Fig. 22.2); that emergency plans should be tested, and that more human engineering studies should be carried out to reduce injuries and deaths within aircraft. The committee also suggested that the FAA develop standards, technical materials, and funding mechanisms to upgrade airport emergency services, and the committee particularly stressed the need for long-range plans on safety and preventive measures.

The committee's report, although exceedingly helpful to local governments and airport operators, unfortunately has not had the desired effect on the concerned federal authorities. There is still a reluctance on the part of the FAA to develop the necessary standards and to require adherence for certification. Nevertheless, the committee is to be commended for its attention to this important problem of safer aircraft and airport services.

SUMMARY

Airports are major centers of community activities. The larger airfields are faced with daily medical emergencies of increasing numbers and occasionally with a major aircraft disaster. A review of the subject has indicated concern on the part of health professionals, the federal government, and other authorities aware of the inadequacies of these services and plans. The character of aircraft accidents are discussed and a check list is provided in the appendix for planners concerned with disaster problems. Since the federal aviation agency is now required to certify airports and their emergency plans and services, more professionalism is required.

REFERENCES

[1] Abelson LC, Star LD, Goldner AS: Twenty years of medical support in aircraft disasters at Kennedy Airport. Aerospace Med 44:560, 1973

[2] Abelson LC, Star LD, Goldner AS: New concepts in casualty treatment and triage at airport disasters. Report at the National Health Resources Advisory Committee, Office of Preparedness, General Services Administration, Chicago, Oct. 11, 1973

[3] Aircraft Accident Report Number L-1011 N310EA, Eastern Airlines Inc., Miami, Fla., Dec. 29, 1972: NTSB-AAR-73-14. Washington, National Transportation Safety Board, 1973

[4] Airport emergency medical facilities and services. Advisory circular No. 150/5210-2, Washington, Federal Aviation Administration, 1964

[5] Airport emergency operations planning. Advisory circular No. 150/5200-10 of July 26, 1968, and change 1 of Sept. 15, 1970. Washington, Federal Aviation Administration, 1968

[6] Annual review of aircraft accident data, U.S. carrier operations calendar year 1969. Report No. NTSM-ARC-71-1, Washington, National Transportation Safety Board, 1971

[7] Bergot GP: Disaster planning at major airports, Aerospace Med 42:449, 1971

[8] Carter JH, Burdge R, Powers SR, Jr., Campbell CJ: An analysis of 17 fatal and 31 non-fatal injuries following an airplane crash, J Trauma 13:346, 1973

[9] Childs JT: Emergency and disaster plans and associated problems concerning major aircraft accidents. Meeting of the National Health Resources Advisory Committee on Airport/Community Emergency Preparedness, Office of Preparedness, General Services Administration, Chicago Oct. 11-12, 1973

[10] Darncer, KL: Short term annual exposure to carbon monoxide and hydrogen cyanide, singly and in combination. FAA Research Task AM-13-73-TOX-24, Washington, Federal Aviation Administration, 1972

[11] Emergency plan. Advisory circular No. 150/5200-17, Washington, Federal Aviation Administration, Department of Transportation Distribution Unit, TAD-484-3, 1972

[12] Guide to organization and operation of airport medical services. Committee on Airport Medical Services, Council on Occupational Health, American Medical Association, JAMA 182-956, 1962

[13] Hays MB: Report of Ad Hoc Committee, California Aviation Safety Council, Airport Medical Facilities, San Fransicso, 1974

[14] Holmbad EC: personal communication, 1969

[15] Jackson FC: Airports: Thresholds of disaster (editorial). J Trauma 10:617, 1970

[16] Jackson FC, Leighton JS, Dornenburg PR, Hammill GP: A comprehensive account of the aircraft accidents at Bradford, Pennsylvania, on December 24, 1968 and January 6, 1969. Unpublished report, Washington, Public Health Service, Division of Emergency Health Services, Department of Health, Education, and Welfare, 1969

[17] Kaetzel PK: Unpublished data, Washington, Public Health Service, Division Emergency Health Services, Department of Health, Education, and Welfare

[18] Mohler SR et al: Aeromedical and human factors aspects of airports. Aerospace Med 42:439, 1971

[19] Morton JH, Cramer LM, Schwartz SI: Emergency care of a major civilian disaster, Arch Surg 89:105, 1964

[20] Physicians' guide to airport medicine. JAMA 199:143, 1967

[21] Report of the National Health Resources Advisory Committee Meeting on Airport/Community Emergency Medical Preparedness (minutes). Chicago, Oct. 11–12, 1973, Washington, Office of Preparedness, General Services Administration, 1974

[22] Ruoff A: personal communication

[23] Schultz T: A critical look at how airport disaster plans work under fire. Today's Health 51:68, 1973

[24] Section 139:55. Emergency plan: Certification and operations: Land airports service CAB—certified air carriers, Federal Aviation Regulations, Washington, Federal Aviation Administration, 1973

[25] Seinbridge VA, Crafft WM, Townsend FM: Medical investigation of aircraft accidents with multiple casualties. J Aviation Med 29:668, 1958

[26] Siegel PV: FAA widens role in education, research. U.S. Med, Jan 15, 1969

[27] Snow CC, LeRoy CH, McFadden EB: A survival study of a modern commercial jet aircraft (Boeing 727) landing accident with subsequent interior fire. Injury and fatality analysis (Salt Lake City, Nov. 11, 1965). Federal Aviation Administration, Civil Aeromedical Institute, Oklahoma City.

[28] Spooner A: The causes of aircraft accidents. A report to Canadian Aeronautics and Space Institute/American Institute of Aeronautics and Astronautics/Cornell-Guggenheim Aviation Safety Center Aviation Safety Meeting, Toronto, Ontario, October 31 to November 1, 1966

[29] White MS: The role of the aviation medical examiner in aircraft disasters. JAMA 196:145, 1966

[30] Zanca P: Types of injuries in airplane crash survivors, South Med J 61:1219, 1968

[31] Zimmerman D: A critical look at airport disaster planning. Today's Health 49:18, 1972.

VI

Special Considerations

Ake Grenvik
Peter Safar

23

Critical Care Medicine Facilities and Personnel

One of the most important recent contributions to the prevention of early death in salvageable individuals has been the application of new knowledge in the biology and technology of critical care medicine (CCM). Experience in the United States and other countries has demonstrated that concentration of critically ill and injured patients in specialized units in major medical centers can reduce mortality and morbidity, enhance teaching and research, and promote efficient utilization of highly trained personnel and expensive complex equipment.

Critical care medicine encompasses the triad of (1) resuscitation; (2) emergency medical care for life-threatening conditions; and (3) inten-

Adapted from Safar, P. et al: Public Health Aspects of Critical Care Medicine and Anesthesiology, Chapter 4 Philadelphia, F. A. Davis Co., 1974.

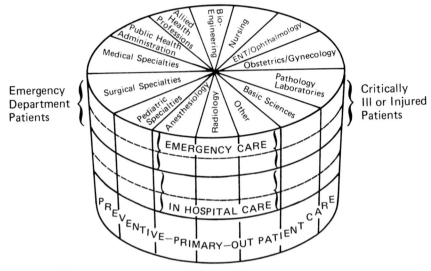

Figure 23.1
The cake represents the body of knowledge and expertise in medicine (pathophysiology and therapeutics) with traditional disciplines (vertical slices) and interdisciplinary programs (horizontal layers).

sive care. Emergency care and critical care are, therefore, part of the same mission, common in kind, but different in scope (Fig. 23.1).

The EMS system is only as strong as its weakest link. The components of the emergency and critical care delivery system are

1. Recognition of the emergency and aid by bystanders (public education)
2. Initiation of the EMS response system (universal emergency telephone number 911, highway phones, radios, communication center)
3. Treatment at the scene by members of the system (police, fire, rescue, ambulance, mobile ICU ambulance, aircraft ambulance)
4. Transportation with life support by members of the system
5. Treatment in emergency department of hospital or in separate advanced life-support facility
6. Treatment in operating room (anesthesia, surgery)
7. Treatment in ICU
8. Organization and communication of 1 and 7
9. Planning, education, and evaluation for 1 and 8
10. Research (laboratory, patient, and health-care delivery research)

The earlier modern life support is applied, the greater is the patient's chance for survival without needing prolonged expensive intensive care and without becoming a financial and emotional burden. In contrast, even the best prehospital care cannot obtain optimal results without properly staffed, equipped, and organized hospital emergency services including ICUs.

Emergency department physicians focus on the 50 million emergency department admissions per year in the United States, which at present consist of about 60% nonemergent cases (seen in the emergency department because of unavailability of primary physicians and/or outpatient clinics); 35% non–life-threatening bona fide emergencies; and 5% (or less) acutely life-threatening emergencies (i.e., critically ill or injured patients.) Critical care medicine physicians (specialists of anesthesiology, emergency medicine, internal medicine, pediatrics, or surgery with special interest, training, and competence in CCM) focus on the less than 5% of emergency department visits with life-threatening conditions and those critically ill or injured patients already in the hospital who have multiple organ system failure and who can benefit from multidisciplinary critical care (Fig. 23.1).

The principal working area for the emergency department physician is the emergency department, and for the CCM physician, it is the ICU. Depending upon individual interest and expertise, both types of physicians should be concerned with the prehospital components (components 1–4) and the coordinating and pioneering of EMS (components 8–10), including community leadership. The primary physician (family physician as well as specialist) may refer the patient into the system, should become a team member or team coordinator within the system depending upon his availability and competence, and may focus on operative care (surgery) and/or noncritical follow-up care.

Prehospital Life Support

Definitions for prehospital life support include (a) basic life support, *i.e.*, advanced first aid taught in the Red Cross course plus cardiopulmonary resuscitation steps A, B, and C, plus features of emergency care that are included in the EMT basic course; and (b) advanced life support, *i.e.*, basic life support plus electrocardiography for recognition of life-threatening arrhythmias, control of arrhythmias with drugs and defibrillation, venous infusion, initiation of spontaneous circulation in cardiac arrest, immediate post-resuscitative care, tracheal intubation, and the use of basic respiratory care equipment. A MICU is designed to provide basic and advanced life support to patients with life-threatening acute illness or injury during transfer to the emergency department, operating room, and/or ICU.

General Intensive Care

General intensive care includes continuous intensive monitoring and life support as well as definitive therapy of patients with critical and acutely life-threatening illness or injury. General intensive care may be of three types.

The first type is advanced intensive medical care, which provides coverage by physicians with special competence in CCM or CCM physician trainees 24 hours a day within the unit. Type two, basic intensive medical care, provides coverage by conventional house officers (*i.e.*, anesthesiology, internal medicine, pediatrics or surgery) or other physicians with basic CCM experience who cover full-time within the unit 24 hours a day. Type three, intensive nursing care, provides only specially trained registered nurses on the spot for coverage within the unit and physicians rounding, writing orders, and being available within the house or on-call at home.

Critical Care Unit

A critical care unit is a specific area of a hospital that provides maximum surveillance and support of vital functions and definitive therapy for patients with acute, but reversible life-threatening impairment of single or multiple vital organ systems. The unit's staff of physicians, nurses, allied health professionals, and others are trained and equipped to provide these services to patients in general medical/surgical ICUs or in special ICUs, such as respiratory care units, coronary care units, neonatal intensive care units, pediatric intensive care units, burn units, and trauma units. Most coronary care units (CCU) are primarily for arrhythmia control by nurses as predirected by physicians.

An emergency department of the hospital is a critical care unit if it is specially staffed and equipped for advanced life support and definitive care of patients with acute illness or injury and if such patients represent a substantial proportion of emergency department admissions.

Intermediate Care

Intermediate care is sometimes necessary for patients who are relatively stable but still require continuous monitoring. These patients do not require devices that assist vital organ functions (*e.g.*, ventilators, hemodialysis machines, assisted circulation devices), since they may never have fully developed an acute life-threatening crisis or are recovering from it.

Historically, ICUs have evolved as postanesthetic/postsurgical recovery rooms in which surgical patients stay as long as they remain critically ill. Premature infants were grouped for infection precaution and temperature control into neonatal ICUs as far back as the 1920s. Respiratory ICUs were started in the early 1950s in Scandinavia for poliomyelitis patients[8] and intoxications[3], and in the late 1950s in the United States, Canada, New Zealand, and other countries. Surgical ICUs for postoperative cardiothoracic patients were also developed in the 1950s. At Baltimore, Maryland hospitals, a multidisciplinary ICU was developed in 1953, the first such unit in the United States to have 24-hour coverage by physicians especially trained in life-support techniques.[14] The life-saving potential of arrhythmia control resulted in the establishment of coronary care units (cardiac care units) in most general hospitals in the United States in the 1960s.

GENERALIZATION AND REGIONALIZATION OF CRITICAL CARE

Continuing advances in medicine and technology coupled with the rapid rise in medical care costs will require the following: (1) nationwide categorization of hospitals (*e.g.*, into four categories according to the criteria established by the American Medical Association); (2) graded patient care in community hospitals and major referral centers ranging from intensive care through intermediate care and routine hospital care to ambulatory (preventive-comprehensive) care; (3) development of regional major medical centers (categories I and II hospitals) for the care of the critically ill and injured strategically located throughout the country and hospitals with intensive nursing care (category III) and transfer facilities with life support to categories II or I hospitals. (Ideally, no patient in the United States should be more than a 1-hour ambulance or aircraft ride from a category III facility; category IV hospitals should provide resuscitation but not necessarily intensive care.)and (4) an efficient and safe emergency transport system with competent technical and professional personnel capable of providing resuscitation and life support to the critically ill and injured patient at the scene and during transportation.

In the United States, at present, approximately 80–90% of acute general hospitals with over 200 beds and 30% of hospitals with less than

Table 23.1. Hospital Staffing in Critical Care Facilities

Categories of hospitals	In house		On call	
	Emergency department	*Hospital*	*Available in < 20 minutes*	*Available in > 20 minutes*
Category I Comprehensive Emergency Medical Center	Registered Nurse Internist Surgeon	Anesthesiologist Internist Pediatrician Surgeon Obstetrician	All specialties and sub specialties	
Category II Major Emergency Hospital	Registered Nurse Physician	Internist Surgeon Nurse Anesthetist	Most specialties including Anesthesiologists	All specialties
Category III General Emergency Hospital	Registered Nurse Physician*	Nurse Anesthetist Physician*	Anesthesiologist Internist Surgeon (Pediatrician)† (Obstetrician)	Most specialties
Category IV Basic Emergency Hospital	Registered Nurse	Nurse Anesthetist	Anesthesiologist Internist Surgeon	

* One physician serves both the emergency department and the total hospital in category III hospitals.
† Parentheses indicate that the availability of the specialty varies from hospital to hospital within a category.

Table 23.2. Types of Intensive Care Units in Different Hospitals

Categories of hospitals	Emergency life support		General intensive care unit			Definitive therapy	
	Basic	*Advanced*	*Intensive nursing care (type 3)*	*Basic intensive med. care (type 2)*	*Advanced intensive med. care (type 1)*	*Basic specialties*	*All specialties*
Category I Comprehensive Emergency Medical Center	Yes	Yes	Yes	Yes Physician	Yes Critical Care Physician	Yes	Yes
Category II Major Emergency Hospital	Yes	Yes	Yes	Yes Physician	No	Yes	No
Category III General Emergency Hospital	Yes	No	Yes	No	No	Yes	No
Category IV Basic Emergency Hospital	Yes	No	(Yes)*	No	No	Yes	No

* Parentheses indicate that the availability varies from hospital to hospital within a category.

291

Table 23.3. Types of Surgical Operations in Different Hospitals

Categories of hospitals	Emergency operations		Elective operations			
	Minor	*Major*	*Minor PS 1–2*	*Major PS 1–2*	*Minor PS 3–5**	*Major PS 3–5*
Category I Comprehensive Emergency Medical Care	Yes	Yes	Yes	Yes	Yes	Yes
Category II Major Emergency Hospital	Yes	Yes	Yes	Yes	Yes	Yes
Category III General Emergency Hospital	Yes	(Yes)†	Yes	Yes	(Yes)	No
Category IV Basic Emergency Hospital	(Yes)	No	Yes	(Yes)	No	No

* PS 1–5 indicate the physical status of patients from 1 (healthy) to 5 (moribund) as classified by the American Society of Anesthesiologists.
† Parentheses indicate that the availability varies from hospital to hospital within a category.

200 beds report having ICUs. Most of these ICUs provide only intensive nursing care, some provide basic intensive medical care, and very few have advanced intensive medical care.

Attempts to give sophisticated care in understaffed and underutilized facilities merely because they have new and expensive equipment are likely to be hazardous for the patient. Patients with life-threatening emergencies should be transported directly to the regional category I/II hospital whenever possible. Experience at the University of Maryland shock-trauma unit shows a threefold increase in long-term survival of critically injured patients when admitted directly to this center, as compared with primary admission to an outlying hospital and delayed transfer to the center.

Patients requiring resuscitation during transportation should be taken to the nearest emergency hospital. If this hospital is not a category I or II facility, the patient's vital function should first be stabilized, but he should be transferred as soon as possible, life support during transportation being provided by a CCM-trained physician, anesthesiologist, internist, or surgeon with EMS experience, nurse anesthetist, respiratory therapist, or especially trained EMT in this order of preference.

The type of ICUs in category I and II hospitals should include at least one general (medical/surgical/coronary) ICU. If arrhythmia control is provided in a separate CCU, it should be adjacent to the general medical/surgical ICU. The care in separate medical and surgical ICUs without automatic consultation (team membership) of various specialists seeing all patients tends to be inferior, and appropriate staffing with nurses is more difficult. Pediatric intensive care for various age groups and neonatal intensive care should be available in regional centers.

Experimental and/or extraordinarily expensive life-support measures requiring highly specialized teams of physicians and nonphysicians (*e.g.,* long-term extracorporeal) oxygenation or assisted circulation; long-term artificial ventilation; preoperative and postoperative care of organ transplantation patients; surgery for severe multiple injuries, including brain, chest, and neonatal emergency surgery) should be concentrated in some but not all categories I and II hospitals and judiciously distributed according to case load.

The type of categorization of hospital emergency and critical care facilities recommended by the authors at this time is based on the AMA's recommendations of 1971[2] and modified locally for Western Pennsylvania, as published in "Guidelines for the Planning and Development of General ICUs in Western Pennsylvania"[7] and in "Public Health Aspects of Critical Care Medicine and Anesthesiology."[12]

Surveying and categorizing hospitals constitute meaningless efforts unless accompanied by a plan based on demographic, geographic, and "need" data; on where certain categories of hospitals must be located; and on what their special roles and interactions should be. Planning is fruitless unless there are means to implement the plan and to evaluate regularly changes in quality of health care.

REGIONAL NEEDS AND DEMANDS FOR ICU BEDS

At present no data are available on the severity of illness (degree of deterioration and physical status) of patients (a) at the time of entering the EMS system; (b) at the time of admission to the hospital's emergency department; and (c) at the time of ICU admission. The proportion of critically ill patients among ICU admissions varies greatly as evidenced by the need for mechanical artificial ventilation, which ranges from 75% for ICU patients at the Presbyterian-University Hospital ICU in Pittsburgh to only 10% in some ICUs of community hospitals in the surrounding area.

Current ICU bed requirements are usually based on demands rather than actual needs. It is difficult to predict future needs because the percentage of ICU beds in relationship to total hospital beds (at present considered arbitrarily as about 2% in general hospitals) will increase with expanded outpatient management of diagnostic and nonoperative care, and the percentage should decrease with improvements in EMS systems. Reducing early mortality at the scene and during transportation, however, may also bring a greater number of critically ill or injured patients to hospitals.

To assist a community in the planning and evaluation of its resources, the following formula is suggested as a guideline for projecting the number of ICU beds needed for a given population. This approach or methodology is designed to be flexible, taking into consideration local conditions, future trends, and regional responsibilities. Projection of bed needs is based on the interrelationship of the various factors that influence future needs. These factors include projected population, admission rate, transfer rate, average length of stay, and desirable average occupancy.

Forecast of ICU Bed Needs

In order to forecast the number of beds needed in the ICU unit, use the following formula:

total population (in thousands)	X	hospital admissions per year per 1,000 population	X	% of hospital patients admitted to ICU	X	average length of stay in ICU (days)

Divide the above figure by the desired average ICU occupancy rate (for instance 75%) times 365 days per year.

For example, the need for a community of 100,000 people with an admission rate of 140 patients per 1,000 inhabitants and an ICU admission rate of 5% of hospital patients with a 5-day average length of stay in the ICU would be 13 ICU beds.

The total population would depend upon the service area involved. The hospital admission rate developed and used for planning purposes on a national and regional basis is approximately 14% of the total population per year to a short-term general hospital. This figure may be used when the actual admission rate is not known. The percentage of hospital patients admitted to the ICUs in Western Pennsylvania is currently slightly less than 5%; in areas where this rate is not known a 5% ICU admission rate may be utilized. The average length of ICU stay in Western Pennsylvania is 5 days. The desired average occupancy rate of 75% represents the percentage of time that available ICU beds are occupied by patients. Availability of vacant beds for unexpected emergencies and maintaining reasonable cost effectiveness plus several years of experience suggest that 75% occupancy is a suitable figure for planning.

ORGANIZATION OF INTENSIVE CARE UNITS

Concentrating critically ill but potentially salvageable patients with multiple organ failure and those requiring prolonged artificial ventilation in an interdisciplinary ICU or a critical care center (combination of adjacent medical, surgical, and cardiac care units) has patient-care advantages and economic advantages over purely respiratory, medical, surgical, or otherwise fragmented ICU facilities, since most critically ill or injured patients have multiple organ failure of both a medical and a surgical nature. For instance, in one institution, when specialty ICUs were replaced with a single multidisciplinary unit staffed with physicians especially experienced in CCM, mortality from respiratory insufficiency decreased from 30% to 10%, and mortality from myocardial infarction decreased from 30% to 15%.[9]

Pediatric patients benefit from interdisciplinary ICUs for children, but neonatal ICUs should be separate, centralized on a regional basis, and located preferably in large maternity hospitals. Adolescents are probably best admitted to adult general ICUs.

Burn units should be located in category I hospitals with high quality backup services, since electrolyte fluid balance and respiratory care (shock lung, pulmonary burns), as well as asepsis, nursing care, and plastic surgery must be sophisticated. Survival of patients with 50–80% surface burns and pulmonary burns depends greatly upon these measures.

Easily accessible geographic connections and functional links between ICUs, emergency departments, and operating rooms are desirable. Ideally, ICUs should consist of clusters of six to eight single-bed glass-enclosed cubicles in which all patients can be seen from the nursing station.

Development of New ICUs

The development of ICUs should be accomplished in an orderly fashion as follows:

1. Planning by an ad hoc committee that includes members of the medical staff (at least anesthesiologist, internist, and/or pediatrician, cardiologist, infectious disease specialist and surgeon), nursing service, administration, biomedical engineer, and hospital architect (The planning committee should determine the intensive care needs of the hospital and community in cooperation with the local EMS council; determine the types of ICUs and number of beds required; estimate costs and propose a budget; recommend a medical director; recommend a head nurse; determine physician responsibilities, authorities, and coverage; determine number of nurses and nurse/patient ratios; provide technical and engineering support; and recommend appointment of a permanent ICU committee. The permanent ICU committee should design a general policy to be approved by the medical staff and administration. The permanent ICU committee should include at least an anesthesiologist, surgeon, internist, and pediatrician (if indicated) who manage patients with acute life-threatening illness or injuries, the medical director and head nurse of the unit plus members of hospital administration and house staff.)
2. Training staff nurses and physicians (*e.g.*, by sending them to hospitals with existing facilities and teaching programs in critical care)
3. Recommending the design and equipment of the unit
4. Opening the ICU with basic staff

5. Developing specific standards for monitoring and life-support techniques
6. Training allied health personnel (respiratory therapists, physiotherapists, and others)
7. Organizing continuing education for physician trainees, staff physicians, and nurses
8. Developing systems for record-keeping, statistical analysis, and review of results
9. Developing full-time physician specialist coverage from various disciplines
10. Fostering research (at least making attempts to evaluate quality of care on the basis of outcome)

The smooth functioning of an ICU depends upon organization, well-defined responsibilities and authorities, and standardization of certain procedures (*e.g.*, cardiopulmonary resuscitation, respiratory care including mechanical ventilation, care of the intubated and tracheotomized patient, humidification, control of inspired O_2 and CO_2 concentration, and respiratory monitoring; recording blood gas values and other important variables; arrhythmia control in the absence of a physician; cardiovascular catheterization and catheter management; general care of the unconscious patient; prevention and control of infections; temperature control including deliberate hypothermia; central nervous system monitoring; and determination and certification of brain death).

PHYSICIAN RESPONSIBILITY AND COVERAGE

Medical Director

Responsibilities for medical care will depend upon local circumstances. The Society of Critical Care Medicine (SCCM) and the JCAH recommend that every ICU have a medical director. He should be chosen on the basis of experience, competence, interest, and availability rather than specialty affiliation. He should have completed residency training in a major clinical specialty and have acquired advanced skills and knowledge in life-support techniques and patient monitoring. If and when certification of "special competence in critical care medicine" becomes available, it is recommended that the ICU medical director display such competence.

In a category I hospital, he should be geographic full-time and devote the majority of his time to the unit. In a category II hospital he may be part-time. He should be responsible to the staff for patient care matters and to the hospital director for administrative matters. One or more codirectors of the ICU whose primary specialties may be distinct from that of the director may share full-time supervision as well as responsibility for teaching and patient care.

The medical director or his designate should approve all admissions and discharges, be responsible for monitoring, resuscitation and life support, and insure that patient care involving multiple services is coordinated. He should have the right to request consultation from other physicians or services and determine which patients will require isolation. He is responsible for administration and education in the unit, which include proposing the annual budget, supervising record-keeping, and evaluating care.

In specialized intradepartmental ICUs it may be possible for every patient admitted to be transferred to the service of the ICU medical director and his house staff, with the admitting physician becoming the consultant.

In multidisciplinary ICUs the complexity of modern critical care makes it unlikely that one person will be competent in all its aspects. Therefore, continuous surveillance and management of patients should be provided by a team of CCM physicians of various disciplines experienced in CCM, plus nurses and allied health personnel. The team should include the patient's personal physician, the director of the ICU or his designate, and a number of specialists, and it should have a team coordinator—not a dictator.

Team Coordinator

A team coordinator with ultimate authority and responsibility for the patient's general care is essential. The patient's personal physician could retain responsibility for his patient's general care and coordination of the team, provided he is available at all times for guidance of the team. If not, he should delegate this role temporarily to a specialist (at least a senior resident) who is available and familiar with critical care or to the ICU director and his staff. The patient's personal physician should remain a member of the team to insure continuity. The coordinator could be that team member who is most experienced in managing the patient's predominant problem. Ideally, all orders should be channeled through a member of the unit's full-time staff or a physician trainee assigned full-time to the unit. Other options would include general orders by the admitting physician who acts as team coordinator, respiratory orders by the full-time ICU physician, and emergency orders by any physician. General and specific care orders in a category III ICU should be written by the patient's primary admitting physician, and nonmedical staff should carry out emergency measures according to standing orders. Because of the traditional possessiveness of the primary physician specialist in the health care system of the United States, patient-care authority has evolved in our general ICUs and in many others according to the following compromise:

Orders are written jointly by the admitting physician (or his house officer) and the ICU fellow. The ICU director and his full-time fellows are automatically involved as team members in the care of all patients and are responsible for life-support monitoring, cardiopulmonary resuscitation, administration, and teaching. Automatic team membership involves more than being a consultant, since the latter must wait until called upon (which may be too late), and he may not be permitted to assume responsibility for any phase of the management. Attending staff and mature house staff of various disciplines have collaborated well in this voluntary team system, but immature and inexperienced house staff sometimes fail to collaborate.

To provide optimum care to the patient and insure efficient operation of the unit, it is advisable to develop a list of consultants in neurology, bronchoesophagology, neurosurgery, orthopedic surgery, infectious diseases, renal and metabolic diseases, radiology, and psychiatry. Such specialists should manifest an interest in applying their specific skills to patients with life-threatening illness and injuries and work cooperatively with members of the unit's staff.

Physicians who provide 24-hour coverage in ICUs should be competent in CCM. Ideally, they should have at least 2 years of approved postgraduate training. Care of the critically ill by inexperienced house staff or by physicians who do not personally (or through experienced designates) remain with the patient should be strongly discouraged.

In category I hospitals, 24-hour coverage within the general ICU should be provided by CCM physicians (trainees or staff men) who are responsible to the director of the ICU, and the CCM physicians should be assigned full-time to the unit without responsibilities in other areas of the hospital.

In category II ICUs, house officers covering general intensive care should also be responsible to the ICU medical director, but they may have less advanced training and experience than the CCM physician trainees or CCM staff physicians in the category I ICU.

In category III ICUs, the primary admitting physician retains responsibility for general care of patients. He should delegate responsibility for ongoing life support and emergency services to nonphysician personnel who act according to standing orders. He should also delegate responsibility for special problems that are beyond his competence to consultants, including the ICU medical director.

It is important that final responsibility for ICU patient care reside with the physician who provides continuous patient observation, who is aware of the patient's overall problems, and has acquired the most experience in CCM.

CCM PHYSICIAN EDUCATION

Manpower Needs

Job opportunities for physicians with special expertise in CCM are ample in traditional departments but are few for autonomous interdisciplinary ICU directors, in spite of JCAH and SCCM recommendations. There are about 1,400 acute general hospitals with over 200 beds in the United States. With an average need of at least one CCM director and one codirector for each hospital's general ICU (24-hour in-house coverage helped by additional physicians), about 2,800 CCM experienced, trained, and committed physicians are needed in the United States now. However, there are probably not many more available than the 300 members of the SCCM. Fewer than 10 CCM fellowship training programs, which approach SCCM education guidelines, trained only 40–50 CCM physicians in 1972–1973. Therefore, such programs should be expanded. In a recommendation for the federal Emergency Medical Services Systems Act, Safar recommended in testimony on behalf of the EMS Systems Act (PL 93–154) that the government provide about $4 million per year for 10 years for CCM physician fellowship training stipends, another $4 million annually for 10 years for emergency department physician training and an additional $10 million per year for 10 years to support EMS–CCM centers for education and research.

At the University of Pittsburgh, we have developed educational objectives separately for medical students, traditional residents, emergency physicians, and CCM physicians in terms of knowledge, skills, experience, ability, and attitude.

Medical Students

Most medical schools have inadequate education programs in resuscitation, emergency care, and intensive care. Only one-third of the medical schools in the United States and Canada offer a formal emergency medical care course. Most are conducted by the department of surgery, are focused on trauma, and are limited to Emergency Department experience. Between 1963 and 1973, at the University of Pittsburgh a combined emergency and CCM program evolved, which is coordinated by a multidisciplinary faculty committee. First-year students receive a 20-hour emergency care course, second-year students receive cardiopulmonary resuscitation (A–D) and respiratory insufficiency instruction, third-year students receive an obligatory 3-week clerkship in CCM (modified from the former anesthesiology clerkship), and fourth-year students have a 9-week elective available to them.

Traditional Disciplines

Although some critical illnesses are covered well by traditional specialists and their house staff (*e.g.*, cardiology/cardiac care unit, nephrology/renal unit, cardiac surgery, and neurosurgery), experience has shown that most traditional residencies, including anesthesiology, medicine, pulmonary diseases, cardiology, pediatrics, surgery, surgical subspecialties, and obstetrics/gynecology, do not prepare graduates adequately for modern care of the critically ill or injured patient with multiple organ failure. An AMA conference recommendation was that CCM training by full-time assignment to teaching ICUs should be available to all residents of traditional clinical disciplines.[4] This training should be obligatory for anesthesiology and emergency physician training programs. Making it mandatory for all clinical specialty residents would be unrealistic because of the limitations of ICU facilities and number of patients available.

CCM Physician Specialist's Fellowship Program

Such a program was started at the University of Pittsburgh in 1963 with the objective of training physicians who would staff and lead general ICUs in community and teaching hospitals. The CCM physician is a traditional specialist (Fig. 23.1, vertical slice) with additional special interest and training in cardiopulmonary resuscitation, life support, CCM organization, and education (Fig. 23.1, thin horizontal slice). He brings special expertise in supportive care, *i.e.*, in the maintenance of vital organ system homeostasis when auto-regulation fails. He is both a specialist and a generalist. He is a generalist because of his interest in patients with multiple organ failure, even though he is involved in their management only in the life-threatening phase. The horizontal stratification of emergency and critical care medicine is in keeping with present public pressure for more comprehensive, rather than specialized, disease-oriented practice.

The CCM physician needs a base specialty because CCM is not a recognized specialty at this time, because he needs in-depth scientific background in a traditional discipline to function as a team member, and because full-time clinical practice in critical care is probably too demanding to be tolerated for an entire lifetime.

The University of Pittsburgh CCM Fellowship Program is flexible to meet the needs of physicians with different specialty backgrounds. Their basic experience is in the general ICU. Fellows selectively rotate through cardiology, nephrology, neonatology, EMS including mobile ICU, and research. One-year fellows are encouraged to participate in clinical research, 2-year fellows in full-time laboratory, clinical, or health-care delivery research. Admission to the fellowship requires at least 2 years of postgraduate training in a base specialty. The fellowship year is approved as the elective year within the 3–4-year residency programs in anesthesiology, medicine, pediatrics, and surgery.

Between 1963 and 1973, 62 CCM fellows were trained in the University of Pittsburgh program. Most of them rotated for 1 year, and most of them were anesthesiologists. There is increasing interest in CCM among nonanesthesiologists, however. In 1973–1974, there were nine CCM fellows, seven anesthesiologists, and two internists. In 1974–1975, there were 12 CCM fellows, three of whom were anesthesiologists, two surgeons, two pediatricians, and five internists. The total number of CCM fellows trained by 1975 was 83.

Experience gained from our program helped in developing national guidelines established by SCCM: The objective of training programs in CCM should be to develop physicians who have acquired the knowledge, skills, experience, judgment, and attitudes for optimal care of critically ill and injured patients; who will provide leadership in the team approach to CCM; and who will function as directors of critical care units and programs. For those intending an academic career, sufficient background for teaching and research is mandatory and should be included as an integral part of an extended program. While CCM fellowship programs should be academically strong, competition between CCM fellows and residents of traditional specialties for experience in treating patients may make nonuniversity hospital ICUs also desirable places for CCM fellows to acquire such clinical experience. The period of training should be flexible and individualized considering previous education, in order to accomplish proficiency and career goals. A minimum of 2 years should be considered for those who intend CCM as a primary career. However, if several years of previous experience in a clinical discipline include guided management of critically ill patients, a CCM fellowship of 1 year may be considered adequate. While emergency and CCM physicians focus on a temporal phase in the patient's overall course, trainees must also be encouraged to learn about the phases preceding and following the patient's emergency department and ICU stays, both for individual patient care and for understanding all components of the system.[15]

Even with intensification of emergency and CCM training within medical schools and conventional residencies, traditional specialists are unlikely to sustain their emergency and CCM experience, since they are not involved in large enough numbers of appropriate cases. In addition, rapid progress in knowledge and technology may be beyond their ability or willingness to assimilate. Further, they may not be able to provide 24-hour life support (titrated care), especially if this schedule prevents them from practicing their base specialties (rounding type of care), or they may lack ability and training to look after education, budgets, organization, administration, quality control of life support, and links with the community, which would not necessarily prevent them from providing care. Finally, they may be unable to innovate and do research in CCM.

In teaching hospitals, CCM physicians suffer from rivalries between departments, specialties, and house staff. In community hospitals, emergency department and CCM physicians seem to complement traditional specialists well. We have recommended combined training of emergency and critical-care physicians in the form of a residency in emergency medicine followed by a fellowship in CCM, primarily for the 24-hour staffing of emergency departments and ICUs in small, non-teaching community hospitals by groups of such specialists.

At an AMA workshop,[11] an evaluation and approval system of CCM fellowships and "certification of special competence in CCM" was recommended as a cooperative venture of the American boards of anesthesiology, medicine, pediatrics, and surgery (and emergency medicine if and when approved as a specialty) and SCCM. Candidates for "special competence in CCM examinations" should be physicians who have passed one of the base specialty board examinations and who have completed an approved CCM fellowship training in addition to the base specialty training. Certification in CCM should be granted by an interdisciplinary body, for instance, the American Board of Medical Specialties.

The following is a checklist for establishing objectives for physician education in CCM. Categorizing requirements as "advanced," "basic," and "not required" is suggested for medical students, for CCM fellows, and for residents in anesthesiology, medicine, pediatrics, surgery, obstetrics/gynecology, surgical specialities, family medicine, and emergency medicine.

Knowledge

First-aid
Emergency medical care
EMS delivery system
Pathophysiology of acute death
Cardiopulmonary resuscitation
Vital organ failure

Respiratory failure
Central nervous system failure
Renal failure
Gastrointestinal-hepatic failure
Circulatory failure

Skills

Cardiopulmonary resuscitation
Airway care, oxygenation,
    ventilation without
    tracheotomy tube
Tracheal intubation, care of
    intubated patient
Cricothyrotomy, transtracheal
    insufflation
Tracheotomy
Therapeutic bronchoscopy
Respiratory care and monitoring
Mechanical ventilation
Inhalation and aerosol therapy
Chest physiotherapy
Blood gas determinations
Acute laboratory techniques
Venous catheterization, arterial
    puncture
Venous cut-down
Arrhythmias
Fluid-electrolyte, acid-base
    balance
Intravenous alimentation
Bleeding/clotting pathology

Temperature control
Infection control
Intoxications
Psychiatric emergencies
Psychological CCM problems
Legal/ethical problems
Current education methods and
    evaluation
Central venous catheterization
Arterial catheterization
Pulmonary artery catheterization
Treatment of shock
Massive venous infusion
Gastric drainage
Bladder drainage
Pleural drainage
Pericardial drainage
Hypothermia
Special central nervous system
    monitoring
Determination of brain death
Instrumentation technology
CCM equipment evaluation

Experience

CPR attempts: team member
CPR attempts: team leader
Multidisciplinary ICU:
    team member

Multidisciplinary ICU:
    team leader
Operating room anesthesia
CCU/cardiology

Dialysis unit/nephrology
Pediatric multidisciplinary ICU
Neonatal ICU/neonatology
Newborn resuscitation
Emergency department

Community EMS/
 mobile ICU ambulance
CCM laboratory research
CCM patient research
CCM health-care delivery research

Special Capabilities

Administration
 Budget preparation, personnel
 management procedures,
 manual preparation, policies
 preparation
Data acquisition and processing

Teaching (cardiopulmonary
 resuscitation, emergency care,
 intensive care)
Planning of community programs
Evaluation of teaching and service
 programs

Attitudes

Community service oriented
Data-oriented
Action-oriented

Team-oriented
Diplomatic
Compassionate

NURSING SERVICE FOR ICUs

Nursing services provided to intensive care patients should be under the direction of a professionally qualified head nurse who is competent in both clinical nursing and administration. The individual selected must have the ability to organize, coordinate, and evaluate the ICU nursing service on a full-time basis.

These functions would include (1) the design and formulation of nursing policies, procedures, functions, and standards of care; (2) the establishment of criteria for staffing and policies regarding staffing; (3) the provision of nursing coverage and teaching personnel; (4) the supervision of nursing care within the unit; and (5) the development of the complete teaching program.

For staffing, a sufficient number of properly trained registered nurses who have demonstrated abilities in problem-solving and developed specialized skills in critical care nursing must be on duty at all times to provide high quality nursing care. The basic average nursing requirement for general ICUs is one registered nurse for every two patients.

Special consideration should be given to patients whose life-support system is not yet stabilized. They require one registered nurse per patient, but it may not always be possible to meet this requirement. To provide true intensive care in such situations, allied health personnel (*e.g.*, licensed practical nurses, nursing assistants, respiratory therapists) may give bedside care within their fields of training. There must be such a "baby sitter" (not necessarily a nurse) at all times for every patient who is not stabilized and every patient requiring mechanical ventilation. One experienced ICU nurse is also required as a team leader for every 2–3 patients. Monitoring techniques should not distract nurses away from bedsides.

Each registered nurse must be able to demonstrate the ability to plan, implement and evaluate the quality of nursing care and to supervise other personnel who may provide nursing-type care not requiring the skill and judgment of a registered ICU nurse.

Training of ICU nurses should include an orientation course, in-service training, and critical care nursing courses.

Orientation. In addition to general hospital orientation, intensive care nurses should have a 6-week ICU orientation course including both theory and clinical application.

In-service training. In-service training in an ICU should be coordinated by a "clinical specialist" whose responsibility is staff development. The head nurse should round daily or at least every other day with the unit's director or codirector, and weekly patient-oriented conferences should be held for all ICU nurses.

Courses. Category I and II hospitals should arrange a critical care nursing course at least twice a year. This course should be made available to clinical specialists and ICU nurses from category III and IV hospitals in the area so that they may become knowledgeable about new diagnostic, monitoring, and therapeutic techniques to facilitate the organization of similar courses at their own hospitals.

Policies for ICU nursing care should be contained in a manual that includes nursing philosophy and objectives, functions and guidelines defining criteria for staffing assignments, admissions, discharges, transfers, definitive therapy, equipment, emergencies, nursing procedures, and general standards of care. Policies for medical management are particularly important for category III ICUs where physicians are not always present.

Registered nurses in an ICU (particularly category III) must be trained to perform according to standing orders and procedures, as described in the ICU nursing manual on cardiopulmonary resuscitation.

These procedures include defibrillation and administration of antiarrhythmic drugs, emergency tracheal intubation, ECG interpretation, arterial and venous puncture, I-V catheter insertion, I-V therapy, peritoneal dialysis, isolation techniques, care of comatose and convulsing patients; and selected techniques in respiratory care.

There should also be standing orders for nonemergency situations regarding patient monitoring, laboratory blood work, daily weighing, chest x-ray examinations, I-V fluid administration, and routine sampling of tracheobronchial secretions for cultures and sensitivity tests. Further, nursing standards of care should be established for patients with acute myocardial infarction, acute respiratory failure, acute renal failure, brain injury, spinal cord injury, multiple injuries, shock, and gastrointestinal bleeding. Standards should also be established for patients on total parenteral nutrition, during postanesthesia recovery, and for postoperative thoracic surgical, cardiovascular, and neurosurgical patients.

PARAMEDICAL PERSONNEL

Modern intensive care has created a need for a great number of paramedical specialists and technicians of various categories. These include inhalation (respiratory) therapists and technicians, physiotherapists, radiology technologists, laboratory technicians, biomedical equipment technicians, social workers, unit managers (administrators), bacteriology technicians, physiologists, computer scientists, programmers, computer technicians, and EMTs. With today's rapid development of new therapeutic methods, including on-line computerized monitoring, use of artificial organs, and extracorporeal circulation, one must anticipate that the number of new and conventional types of paramedical specialists in ICUs will continue to increase.

Respiratory Therapist

By far the most important paramedical specialist in the ICU is the respiratory therapist. In contrast to the prevalent development of respiratory therapists as "IPPB treatment technicians" the AMA-approved school of respiratory therapists of the University of Pittsburgh was started in 1962 because of the obvious need for therapists in cardiopulmonary resuscitation and ICU work for which they are invaluable. They also participate in training ICU nurses and EMTs. This CCM orientation of respiratory therapists has proved particularly valuable in small community hospitals that do not have 24-hour physician staffing.

307

Many of the more than 200 graduates from the Pittsburgh School of Respiratory Therapy are now staffing community hospitals of the area. Following the regulations of the American Registry of Inhalation Therapists many schools of respiratory therapy have become affiliated with community colleges. However, we are concerned about the shift of emphasis under college rule from clinical hospital training and from direction by physicians.

ANCILLARY STAFF

An electrical safety officer should be appointed to provide preventive maintenance of all electric equipment and systems in the unit.

A clerk typist should assist the head nurse during daytime shifts to facilitate efficient patient and administrative record-keeping, purchase orders, telephone calls, and physician page calls.

If the hospital utilizes unit managers, there should be a separate ICU manager who is responsible for control and ordering of supplies and equipment, as well as coordination of other administrative functions, including budgets.

ICU VISITORS

There should be an adjacent waiting room for ICU patients' relatives with a receptionist who will communicate between ICU patients, personnel, and attending physicians. Visiting times should be flexible if possible, but only two visitors should be permitted for each patient at a time. Visitors should wash hands and put on gowns before entering the ICU. Further, there should be a brochure available in the waiting room that explains ICU functions to relatives.

PHYSICAL DESIGN AND EQUIPMENT OF ICUS

Architectural plans of existing critical care facilities should be carefully reviewed before determining the design of new ICUs to insure maximum surveillance and easy access to the patient.

Since small ICUs become uneconomical and impractical because of fluctuations in occupancy, it is recommended that a minimum of six beds be provided. If a hospital requires less than six intensive care beds, these may be combined with coronary care beds or postoperative recovery beds. Clusters of six to eight beds and one central nursing station for each cluster are recommended if needs are greater than eight intensive care beds. Individual isolation rooms must be provided for patients with communicable diseases, as well as for patients in reverse isolation.

Cubicles can be used interchangeably to isolate patients in need of quiet, those with noisy or otherwise disturbing behavior, those with infections (conventional isolation), and those who need to be isolated to avoid infections (reverse isolation). Normal working facilities should be ample. Open areas, which are becoming obsolete, should have partitions between beds to provide privacy and minimize spread of infection by contact. Recommended floor space is at least 150 sq ft per bed in open multiple bed areas and 200 sq ft per bed in isolation cubicles.

Support space for storage of equipment, utility rooms, x-ray facilities, and an acute care laboratory should also be planned. Minimum ancillary rooms for a category III ICU include an adjacent family-lounge waiting room; offices for the ICU director, his secretary, and the head nurse; a personnel lounge within the unit; and equipment storage space about 100 sq ft per bed. Category I and II ICUs should be planned to provide an ancillary room for x-ray films, room for deceased patients, an adjacent physician on-call room, and a conference room for consultation and in-service training programs.

Minimum equipment requirements for a category III ICU include the following installations per cubicle/bed: two oxygen outlets, three vacuum outlets, a compressed air outlet, eight electric outlets, a sink, central monitoring and recording devices, and air conditioning. Category I and II ICUs should meet these minimum requirements and should also be equipped with a computer connection.

In category I and II hospitals, x-ray facilities should be sufficiently comprehensive to provide nearly all of the patient's x-ray requirements. Since patients requiring constant monitoring and life-support equipment can seldom be transported out of the unit to a routine x-ray facility, improved patient care and lower mortality should be achieved by locating x-ray facilities in the unit. In category III and IV hospitals, the minimum requirement is a portable x-ray machine for the intensive care unit.

There is no evidence at this time that use of computers in ICU monitoring decreases morbidity, mortality, or cost, mainly because there are no useful cost-effectiveness studies. Physiologic titration of care is enhanced by on-line computerized monitoring, but the great impact may not come until computerized techniques "close the loop" from sensors to therapy (servo-controlled life support). Beds in the ICU must be adjustable for various positions, and the patient must be accessible from the vertex.

Laboratory determinations for a category III ICU must be made available 24 hours a day either from the hospital's central laboratory or from an ICU stat laboratory. The determinations include blood PO_2, PCO_2, pH (within 5 min); hemoglobin/hematocrit and other basic hematologic tests; electrolytes in serum and urine; glucose in blood and urine; and future basic determinations. In addition to these minimal requirements, laboratories in category I and II ICUs should provide analyses of oxygen saturation/content in blood, serum albumin and globulin, serum and urine osmolality, oxygen consumption, clotting parameters, microscopy for sputum bacteriology, and future advanced determinations.

Crash Cart Equipment and Drug Requirements

The following recommendations for equipment and drug requirements for life support were made by the American Heart Association/National Research Council and are applicable to the hospital crash cart.[1]

Respiratory management. For airway management and artificial ventilation, all life-support units should be equipped with the following:

Oxygen supply (two E cylinders) with reducing valves capable of delivering 15 liters/min and with mask and reservoir bag
Steiner spray cannula
Mask for mouth-to-mask ventilation
Oropharyngeal airways
S-tube (optional)
Laryngoscope with blades (curved and straight, adult and infant) and extra batteries and bulbs
Assorted adult-size (cuffed) and child-size (uncuffed) endotracheal tubes with stylet and 15 mm/22 mm adaptors
Syringe with clamp or plastic two-way or three-way valve for endotracheal tube cuffs
Acceptable bag-valve-mask (adult, child, and infant), with provisions for 100% oxygen ventilation
Bite-blocks
Adhesive tape (1 and 0.5 in.)
Suction (preferably portable), with catheters sizes 6 to 16 and Yankauer-type suction tips
Nasogastric tube
Esophageal obturator airway (optional)
Cricothyreotomy set

Circulatory management. To provide adequate management of the circulatory system, all advanced life-support units should be equipped with the following:

Portable defibrillator monitor with ECG electrode-defibrillator paddles or portable DC defibrillator and portable ECG monitor
Portable ECG machine, direct writing, with connection to monitor
Venous infusion sets (micro and regular)
Indwelling venous catheters (regular and special units): catheter outside needle (sizes 14 to 22); catheter inside needle (sizes 14 to 22); CVP catheters
I-V solutions (5% dextrose in water, lactated Ringer's solution)
Cut-down set
Sterile gloves
Urinary catheters
Assorted syringes and needles, stopcocks, and venous extension tubes
Intracardiac needles
Tourniquets, adhesive, disposable razor, and similar items
Thoracotomy tray

Essential drugs. All life-support units must have the following drugs available:

Sodium bicarbonate (prefilled syringes, 50 ml ampules, or 500 ml 5% bottles)
Epinephrine (prefilled syringes)
Atropine sulfate (prefilled syringes)
Lidocaine (Xylocaine prefilled syringe)
Morphine sulfate
Calcium chloride or calcium gluconate

Useful drugs. These drugs are recommended for hospital and nonhospital life-support units:

Aminophylline	Methylprednisolone (Solu-Medrol)
Dexamethasone (Decadron)	Nalorphine HCl
Dextrose 50%	l-norepinephrine (Levophed)
Digoxin (Lanoxin)	Phenylephrine HCl
Diphenhydramine HCl (Benadryl)	(Neo-Synephrine)
Ethacrynic acid	Potassium chloride
Furosemide (Lasix)	Propranolol HCl (Inderal)
Isoproterenol HCl (Isuprel)	Procainamide HCl (Pronestyl)
Lanatoside C (Cedilanid)	Quinidine HCl
Meperidine HCl (Demerol)	Succinylcholine chloride
Metaraminol (Aramine)	Tubocurarine chloride

Modern critical care techniques necessitate a more vigorous electrical safety program than in regular patient units. This program, supervised by the electrical safety officer, should include necessary electric equipment maintenance, a program for regular checking of equipment, heavy duty three-prong plugs on all equipment, regular checking of defibrillator output, analysis of unexplained recorder or monitoring interference, prohibition of electric beds in the ICU, special rules for external pacemakers (only battery-operated pacemakers), and regular documentation of safety testing.

Electrocution hazards should be minimized by following national standards, which call for equipotential grounding plus an isolation transformer for each bed and current leakage no greater than 10μa from any equipment.[10]

The air conditioning/ventilation system according to 1969 standards from the U.S. Public Health Service should provide slightly positive pressure within the ICU, two minimum exchanges of outdoor air, and six minimum total air exchanges per hour. However, experts currently recommend at least 12 exchanges per hour without recirculation.

BOOKKEEPING, MORTALITY, AND COST EFFECTIVENESS

Bookkeeping

The majority of patients admitted to emergency departments and ICUs in the United States do not have a family physician and/or have changed homes several times; thus they do not have a "cradle to grave" data base concerning their health. This often makes emergency and critical care frustratingly crisis-oriented and episodic. Even when a patient or a patient's relative can give a quick history, records on previous encounters with physicians or hospitals may be unobtainable. At times, patients are improperly managed because of the lack of records. Modern computer technology has made it possible to get important health data for each person on a single record, which would be accessible to the person's physician in any phase of the EMS system. Provided confidentiality can be preserved, this method is highly desirable.

Patients transferred between and within hospitals should be accompanied by information on their illnesses or injuries and their treatments. Ambulance and emergency department records, which ideally should be uniform community-wide and state-wide, must become part of the patient's hospital record. Noting exact time, ambulance and emergency department personnel should, whenever possible, record vital signs, observations, actions taken, treatments given, and statements made by witnesses and the patient's relatives.

Mortality and Cost Effectiveness

Intensive care is "expensive care." The prevalent $100 per day charges do not reflect total charges or costs, which amount to $300–$700 per patient day. Cost/benefit ratios in intensive care are difficult to determine. What, after all, is the value of a human life? There are certainly many patients on whom "expensive care" is wasted. In a study by Fairley and associates, 25% of 1700 patients admitted to ICUs required mechanical ventilation.[6] In patients who required this form of treatment for more than 24 hours, the mortality at 1 month was 50%. In another study, Cullen and Briggs categorized severity of illness in ICU patients; 16% of all patients were in the worst category; 52% of these died within 1 month and 67% within 3 months.[5] Obviously, there is an urgent need to develop criteria for better prediction of the chance for survival and "quality of life" after ICU discharge.

The death rate from heart attacks in hospitals throughout the United States was about 30% before the introduction of CCUs. This death rate was reduced to about 25% by the introduction of CCUs, to 15% when specially trained CCU nurses were permitted to defibrillate and give drugs when indicated, and further to about 10% where physician coverage around the clock was provided in addition to coverage by nurses. The incidence of cardiogenic shock seems to be reduced where prehospital arrhythmia control (mobile ICU) is practiced. A further reduction in mortality from cardiogenic shock may occur with sophisticated cardiopulmonary intensive care (including mechanical ventilation and assisted circulation) during coronary angiography and emergency cardiac (coronary) surgical procedures. This care inevitably will make the CCU an interdisciplinary unit. As another example of the benefits of critical care units, the mortality of critically ill newborn infants was reduced by 50% with the introduction of neonatal ICUs.

Establishment of multidisciplinary and respiratory ICUs resulted in similar reductions in mortality, particularly when full-time physician coverage was added to intensive nursing care. Between 1965 and 1973 in our principal adult ICU, while physician coverage has steadily increased, overall mortality has remained about the same, approximately 20% of ICU admissions. Death rates from cardiogenic shock (10%), brain failure (6.6%), and renal failure (1.7%) have changed little. Respiratory deaths have decreased slightly from 3.3% of admissions in 1965–1966 to 2.2% in 1972–1973, while the proportion of patients in critical condition increased as the number of patients with mechanical ventilation increased from 20% to 70% of admission. Mortality of patients who received mechanical ventilation decreased from 49% in 1965–1966 to 30% in 1972–1973.

In our pediatric ICU, total mortality (corrected for the same admission criteria) decreased from 26% of admissions in 1967–1968 to 15% in 1971–1972. At the same time, as incidence of mechanical ventilation increased from 14% to 46%, mortality of patients on mechanical ventilation decreased from 41% to 30%.

We attribute improved salvage in part to full-time physician staffing. In the adult ICU, the staff increased from one fellow in 1963 to five fellows plus two staff physicians in 1972–1973; in the pediatric ICU, the staff increased from no full-time physician in 1965 to one fellow in 1967 and two staff physicians plus three fellows in 1972–1973.

THE FUTURE

As the technology of life support is becoming increasingly complex and expensive, we should learn to judge better the value of critical care on the basis of chances for "quality life" thereafter. This factor should add philosophy and law to the disciplines CCM leaders must become involved in.

Intensive care units in category I hospitals will become increasingly used for complex techniques such as extracorporeal oxygenation and assisted circulation. Patients who will remain for days and weeks in such units will require an increase in space, equipment, intensive monitoring, and specialized personnel.

We need better ways to evaluate the results of the system according to outcome, in terms of mortality, morbidity, and duration and quality of life. Cost effectiveness should be assessed and related to other needs of society. We also need simple methods to measure outcome to assess which specific patient care measures are important in terms of patient results. Such objective criteria can for young physicians be a substitute for experience. Many complicated techniques and new drugs result in an increasing number of iatrogenic complications which fill our ICUs. Objective evaluation of care requires quantitation of input, not only by grouping patients with the same diagnosis but also, and more importantly, according to their degree of deterioration (physical status) at the time they enter the system.

Separate service status within hospitals for emergency departments and ICUs is becoming a pattern and has been recommended by JCAH, American College of Emergency Physicians, SCCM, and other organizations. For administrative matters, emergency department and ICU directors should report to the hospital director, for patient care matters to the medical staff of the hospital, and for academic matters to the director of the emergency and critical care medicine program of the medical school. Separate emergency and/or critical care medicine departments in medical schools may build new barriers. Institutes may be appropriate for primarily multidisciplinary research programs.

In the United States, national recommendations and standards concerning EMS, CCM, and intensive care are adequate and will be periodically updated. Local implementation lags behind, however, since this implementation must include all components of the delivery system. Whether or not CCM will indeed develop in a well-organized and regionalized fashion will largely depend on community and state authority and responsibility in association with the forthcoming national health insurance and delivery program.

Among the various health-care strata (Fig. 23.1), strong support of comprehensive preventive care at one extreme and emergency and critical care at the other will probably save more lives than the support of regular (intermediate organ or disease-oriented) hospital care. Emergency and CCM could become most striking breakthroughs in health-care delivery in the United States, if supported as mission-oriented interdisciplinary programs.

Although moral and legal consideration of "extraordinary" versus "ordinary" means of life support and discontinuance of efforts in critically ill and injured patients in hospitals and particularly in ICUs are beyond the scope of this chapter, we would like to conclude by stressing that resuscitation in the terminal stages of incurable disease is a violation of the individual's right to die with dignity. It is legally appropriate to indicate in the patient's chart, "Do not resuscitate." The human brain should be the "target organ" of modern life-support efforts.

REFERENCES

[1] American Heart Association, National Research Council: Standards for cardiopulmonary resuscitation and emergency cardiac care. JAMA 227:837, 1974

[2] American Medical Association Commission on Emergency Medical Services: Categorization of hospital emergency capabilities. Chicago, American Medical Association, 1971

[3] Clemmesen C, Nilsson E: Therapeutic trends in the treatment of barbiturate poisoning. Clin Pharmacol Ther 2:220, 1961

⁴ Conference on Education of the Physician in Emergency Medicine. Chicago, American Medical Association, July, 1973

⁵ Cullen D, Briggs B: Survival and follow-up results of critically ill intensive care patients (abstr). Crit Care Med 1:114, 1973

⁶ Fairley HB, Schlobohm RM, Singer MM, Lindauer JM: The appropriateness of intensive respiratory care (abstr). Crit Care Med 1:115, 1973

⁷ Grenvik A, Safar P (co-chairmen, Guidelines Task Force): Guidelines for the planning and development of general ICUs in western Pennsylvania. Pittsburgh, Comprehensive Health Planning Association of Western Pennsylvania, 1974

⁸ Ibsen B: The anesthetist's viewpoint on treatment of respiratory complications in poliomyelitis during the epidemic in Copenhagen, 1952. Proc R Soc Med 47:72, 1954

⁹ Kassebaum DG: personal communication

¹⁰ National Fire Protection Association. National Electrical Code, Boston, 1971. Pennsylvania Medical Society, Commission on Emergency Medical Services: Emergency medical and health services: Present status; recommendations for improvement. Pa Med 74:43, 1971

¹¹ Report on the Conference on Education of the Physician in Emergency Medical Care. Chicago, American Medical Association, July, 1973

¹² Safar P, Benson DM, Esposito G, Grenvik A, Sands P: Emergency and critical care medicine—Local implementation of national recommendations. Public Health Aspects of Critical Care Medicine and Anesthesiology. Ed. P Safar. Philadelphia, F.A. Davis Co., 1974, pp. 65-125

¹³ Safar P: Intensive care unit. Anaesthesia (London) 16:275, 1961

¹⁴ Safar P, Grenvik A: Critical care medicine: Organizing and staffing intensive care units. Chest 59:535, 1971

¹⁵ Society of Critical Care Medicine: Guidelines for physician education in critical care medicine. Crit Care Med 1:39, 1973

SUGGESTED READING

American Heart Association: Coronary Care Units (1) and (2). A specialized intensive care unit for acute myocardial infarction. Mod. Concepts Cardiovasc Dis 34:23, 27, 1965

American Society of Anesthesiologists Committee on Acute Medicine: Community-wide emergency medical services recommendations. JAMA 204:595, 1968

Boehler J, Kroesl W: A comprehensive system of trauma services (Austria). Mod Med 40:57, 1972

Boyd DR: A symposium on the Illinois trauma program: A systems approach to the care of the critically injured. (Introduction: A controlled systems approach to trauma patient care). J Trauma 13:275, 1973

General standards of construction and equipment for hospital and medical facilities. HSMHA publication No. 73–4014. Washington, U.S. Department of Health, Education, and Welfare, February, 1969

Grenvik A: Allied health professionals in intensive care. Crit Care Med 2:6, 1974

Holmdahl MH: Respiratory care unit. Anesthesiology 23:559, 1962

Joint Commission on Accreditation of Hospitals: Accreditation manual for hospitals, Hospital Accreditation Program, 1973

Kampschulte S, Safar P: Development of a multidisciplinary pediatric intensive care unit (abstr). Crit Care Med 1:114, 308, 1973

Kirimli B: Equipment selection for ICUs. Hospitals 43:46, 1969

Lown B, Klein MD, Hershberg PI: Coronary and precoronary care. Am J Med 46:705, 1969

O'Donohue WJ, Baker JP, Bell GM, Muren O, Patterson JL: The management of acute respiratory failure in a respiratory intensive care unit. Chest 58:603, 1970

Pennsylvania hospital resources for the care of respiratory disease patients, standards and survey. Philadelphia, Pennsylvania Thoracic Society, 1971

Rogers R (ed): Cardiorespiratory intensive care. Part I. Chest (suppl) 62(2), 1972

Rogers R (ed): Cardiorespiratory intensive care. Part II. Chest (suppl) 62:(5), 1972

Rogers RM, Weiler C, Ruppenthal B: Impact of the respiratory intensive care unit on survival of patients with acute respiratory failure. Chest 62:94, 1972

Safar P: The anesthesiologist as "intensivist." Science and Practice in Anesthesia. Ed. JE Eckenhoff. Philadelphia, J. B. Lippincott, Co., 1965

Safar P, Grenvik A, Kampschulte S, Benson D, Kirimli B, Smith B: Physician education in critical care medicine. Proceedings of the World Congress of Anesthesiologists WFSA, Kyota, Japan, September, 1972, and Annual Meeting of the American Society of Anesthesiologists, (abstr of scientific papers, p. 101) San Francisco, Calif., October 1973

Society of Critical Care Medicine: Guidelines for organizations of critical care units. JAMA 222:1532, 1972

Standards for special care units. Guidelines for organization, staffing, and costs. Mod Hosp 118:83, 1972

Weil M (ed.): Symposium on critical care medicine. Mod Med 39:82, 1971

John M. Howard

24

The American Trauma Society

The American Trauma Society is a volunteer health organization founded for the purpose of preventing accidental injuries and improving the care of the injured. Its membership is open to anyone who is concerned with the problems of trauma—physicians, patients, nurses, friends, and especially the ordinary citizen who himself may become a victim of trauma.

The concept of such a society originated with a small group of surgeons who recognized the need for a centralized effort to combat the growing problem of accidental injuries in this country and decided to do something about it. Over the years, fatalities due to accidental injuries had been steadily rising until they were the leading cause of death in persons from 1 to 37 years of age and the fourth leading cause of all deaths. Despite the tragic toll of trauma, no concentrated attempt had previously been made to establish a national community-wide organization to spearhead the fight against this "neglected disease." The knowledge, skills, and equipment to prevent many accidental deaths and disabilities existed, but the ability to deliver these to the point of need had been lacking. This is the overall objective of the American Trauma Society.

Rather than actually taking care of the patient, the society strives to bring together physicians, the ambulance profession, the insurance industry, safety engineers, public health officials, communication experts, medical organizations, law enforcement and fire protection professionals, teachers, the press, the armed forces, and governmental agencies in a coordinated effort. These concerned groups, working together, can create programs in all spheres of scientific, clinical, and community endeavor that will effectively meet the challenge of trauma.

ORGANIZATION

The physicians who founded the society realized that to an even greater extent than in cancer or heart disease the public must be involved, for they not only control many of the causes of injury but also provide the first line of defense after it occurs. By educating and mobilizing the community their tremendous resources can be utilized.

For this reason the organization is patterned after the American Cancer Society and the American Heart Association, both of whom foster respect and cooperation between members of the medical profession and enormous numbers of lay people working together to achieve common goals.

The American Trauma Society is chartered in the State of Delaware with a tax-exempt status. It has a board of directors, a house of delegates, officers, an executive director, and members from all 50 states, the District of Columbia, and several foreign countries. Among these are whites; blacks; men; women; physicians; nurses; ambulance, police, and fire personnel; farmers; industrialists; senators; governors; lawyers; engineers; publishers; insurance company presidents; educators; ministers; labor leaders; philanthropists; housewives; fathers; and mothers —all of whom have pledged themselves to work at state and national levels.

In addition to the members who contributed financially to help launch the society, anyone is eligible for membership and participation. This is not a closed organization, rather, it welcomes all participants who wish to join the fight against accidental injuries—trauma.

Within the organizational structure, working with the help and guidance of the national society, are the state divisions, each a separately chartered nonprofit corporation. These are subdivided into nonincorporated local county or regional units and their branches. The latter usually encompass a community or a city, the real grass roots of the society. Here the emphasis is on mobilizing community resources and obtaining the financial support necessary for the society's overall operation. All funds raised at the local level are divided between the state society and the national society.

Each division elects members to the house of delegates, which offers consultation and advice to the national board of directors. An effort is made to have the members of all these various groups, regardless of size, divided as equally as is practical between physicians and nonphysicians.

HISTORY

The American Trauma Society traces its beginning to a meeting of the Committee on Shock of the National Research Council in Washington, D.C., in 1964. At that time it was agreed by the surgeons attending the meeting that a two-pronged attack should be launched against trauma: the creation of a National Institute of Trauma within the government's National Institutes of Health, and the formation of an independent, nonprofit health organization to be known as the American Trauma Society.

A concentrated effort was made to assemble the facts necessary to support such action, including the current status of initial care and EMS afforded to the victims of accidental injury. A summary of these deliberations and a number of recommendations designed to reduce accidental death and disability were published in a report in September 1966 by the National Academy of Sciences/National Research Council under the title "Accidental Death and Disability: The Neglected Disease of Modern Society."[1] This official publication called for the creation of an American Trauma Society.

Five years passed before the society was officially activated, but in the interval informal discussions took place wherever surgeons gathered in connection with some phase of trauma or emergency care of the injured. Opinion was unanimous that an urgent need for such an organization existed. Meanwhile a charter and bylaws were drawn up by a steering committee, which was appointed in July 1967, and a year later the American Trauma Society was incorporated in the State of Delaware.

In the meantime endorsement was sought and received from the American Medical Association, the American College of Surgeons, the American Academy of Orthopedic Surgeons, and the American Association for the Surgery of Trauma. The latter three organizations donated funds to help launch the fledgling society, and all four eventually appointed representatives to serve on the board of directors. The National Safety Council was also represented on the board.

During this formative period the American Cancer Society and the American Heart Association offered invaluable advice, while the Ambulance Association of America and the National Ambulance and Medical Services Association joined in lending their support.

At a formal meeting in Philadelphia in December 1971, final steps were taken for the creation of the American Trauma Society. Officers and board members were elected, committees appointed, and a category of "founding members," contributing $100 each, was established to provide the support for initial development.

In February 1972, the society received tax-exempt status and in May 1972, the first meeting of members was held, with 186 attending. Already the zealous efforts of a handful of dedicated Americans was reaping results.

Soon an executive director was recruited, an office staff enlisted, and from then on the concept of the American Trauma Society spread rapidly across the country. State divisions were formed and chartered by the parent organization, local units established, and the American Trauma Society was well on its way to being a viable and extremely valuable organization working for the health and safety of mankind.

GOALS

The present goals of the American Trauma Society are wide-ranging and will no doubt be modified with the experience and growth of the organization. But the basic purpose should remain the same—to mobilize interest, community forces, funds, people, and programs to understand and support the injured, so that trauma will no longer be "the neglected disease of modern society."

The goals of the society are

1. To educate the public in better organization for the care of injured victims. To develop a community council in every county or community to organize EMS.
2. To improve communications systems by providing a 911 system, a central ambulance dispatcher, and two-way voice communica-

tions between ambulances and hospitals, fire, and police services. To abolish the day of the unexpected arrival of the ambulance at the hospital!

3. To improve ambulance services by professionalizing personnel and redesigning ambulances and equipment to move definitive life-support capability forward to the scene of the accident.
4. To improve emergency departments and to insure that comprehensive hospital emergency facilities are available to all people, 24 hours a day, 7 days a week.
5. To train doctors, nurses, and ambulance personnel in the specialized techniques of emergency care of the injured victim.
6. To support research into better treatment of the major causes of fatal injuries: head and spinal injuries, burns, infections, failure of kidneys and lungs, and the multiple contributing factors.
7. To systematically gather facts on the causes of injuries in each community and apply this knowledge to their prevention across the breadth of the community. To make "hospitalized injury" a disease that can be reported to the state health department.
8. To register and follow up the injured victim throughout his lifetime to determine the late or prolonged effects of trauma.

REFERENCES

[1] Accidental death and disability: The neglected disease of modern society, Washington, Superintendent of Documents, U.S. Government Printing Office, 1966

Martin D. Keller

25

Emergency Health Care: Opportunities for the Health Planner

Emergency medical services encompass a broad range of health care elements that might best be described as a subsystem for coping with unscheduled events in the health-care system. For the health planner, this aspect of health care affords an approach to many major social concerns in health as well as in other vital community planning sectors. It was largely through recognition of these opportunities for the planner that the Graduate Program in Health Policy and Planning of the Ohio State University focused on this area for research and student experience. As we looked into the characteristics of the emergency health-care delivery system, it became apparent that this system was an important barometer of the overall health-care system. It highlighted the interrelationship between the health services and other critical areas of community activity and the gaps in such services. Data collected in various components of the emergency health-care system were useful in coming to grips with the distribution and determinants of many important health conditions. They also revealed the manner in which many affected individuals find their way into the health-care system.

Partly as a result of publicity in the mass media and partly as a result of individual and group concerns, there is public awareness of the need for EMS. Federal, state, and local funding organizations are more and more impelled to respond to this public expression of interest and concern. There are few programs in which a planning agency can have such ready public backing. It is also evident from programs that have been undertaken that it is feasible to introduce changes in the system that can demonstrate benefit in a relatively short period of time. From the start of implementation of a plan to augment emergency services, changes in access to service and in the overall quality can generally be demonstrated in a period of 1 or 2 years. There are few health programs in which desirable change can be so readily demonstrated in so short a period. Of course the impact of investments in emergency service on health outcome requires more sophisticated investigation and probably will take more time. It appears that planning agencies can gain credibility and support, however, in their communities through involvement in EMS planning and thus acquire the recognition needed for successful planning and implementation of other, less visible health-service programs.

REGIONALIZATION OF HEALTH CARE

One of the key issues in health planning is regionalization. There is perhaps no other aspect of health care in which the need for regionalization is so apparent as in emergency services. The requirements of reasonable response time and the constraints of distance in relation to hospital location pose clear indicators for the development of service regions. In general, small communities and rural areas have difficulty in developing effective emergency medical services of their own, and they require cooperative programs with nearby communities. In addition, two of the basic services in any community, transportation and communication, are directly related to emergency medical services. In planning community development, in general, emergency planning contributes vital information for communication systems and transportation plans that allow efficient movement to centers of treatment. In fact the entire matter of crisis intervention is part of emergency planning, and is closely bound up with the ability of citizens to live in various types of communities with a sense of security in the knowledge that critical services are available rapidly and effectively.

COMMUNITY PARTICIPATION

Emergency planning also offers an important opportunity to involve the public and private sectors in cooperative programs. In many communities there is an array of services, tax-supported ambulance squads, private ambulance companies, and hospitals as quasi-public organizations. The emergency room door is an important interface between the community and the hospital. In some areas, where special programs of helicopter rescue have been introduced, there is also an interaction between civilian and military agencies. All of these sectors in society have been brought together in organizations most frequently termed EMS advisory councils. Such organizations serve as forums for the interaction of many different individuals and groups concerned with a wide array of medical needs and services. There is a growing tendency for such organizations to be associated with area-wide health-planning agencies, who also supply the working staff for the advisory councils. This association affords the planner with access to influential persons and groups, whose interests and support may go far beyond the traditional emergency services.

UTILIZATION OF EMERGENCY DEPARTMENTS

In most emergency departments, 60–90% of the individuals seeking medical care would be appropriately classified as requiring primary medical care rather than emergency care. It becomes evident that emergency departments, for the most part, are 24-hour primary care clinics with varying capabilities of dealing with truly urgent problems. Many ambulance services are actually medical transport services, with a relatively small proportion of cases actually requiring emergency care. Experience has shown that emergency communication systems soon become generalized crisis-call channels. People utilize the same communication links for calling police, fire, emergency medical care, poison control, suicide prevention, and a variety of other specific and nonspecific services for assistance in situations that generate anxiety. With respect to hospital emergency departments, the tendency to engage in primary care has been further enhanced by the development of medical groups that contract with the hospital to offer emergency services. There is an economic incentive to serve as many patients as possible. Although this system offers many opportunities, it also poses some serious problems. Patients go to emergency departments because of convenience, inability to obtain close appointments with local physicians, or through habit. In some situations they expect to get better care at the hospital. The emergency department services tend to be expensive, however, charging both for the use of the emergency room and for the physician service. They are often entirely episodic, with little or no attempt at follow-up. Even when referrals are made to community physicians, evidence has shown that these are frequently not followed and that the same problem of obtaining a close appointment deters the patient. For the most part, emergency department physicians are reluctant to bring patients back to the emergency room for follow-up. Consequently, there tends to be little continuity of care and little attempt to evaluate the overall health needs of the patient. Since fairly substantial segments of the population in many areas use the emergency department as their main entry point into the health system, they get practically no continuity of care.

The trend to increasing utilization of the emergency departments would indicate a need for restructuring of the task of the emergency department in relationship to the overall health-care delivery system. Attempts have been made to employ a "follow-up clerk" in the emergency department to check on the status of the patient at an appropriate time after the visit and to further emphasize the need for medical care beyond the services of the emergency department. This type of clerk or a health professional may also serve to obtain information regarding the outcome of emergency services. Most often, the emergency department completely loses touch with the patient, and there is no feedback of information regarding the efficacy of emergency treatment.

Health Surveillance Centers

Emergency departments may also serve as community health surveillance centers. Early information may be obtained regarding injuries caused by consumer products. In fact, a consumer product surveillance program has been instituted in a number of emergency departments around the country. This program can be readily augmented to serve regional and national needs. In general, data obtainable in emergency departments can help to delineate the urgent medical care needs of the community and the types of patients that bypass other sources of health care. Both of these are clearly necessary information for the assessment of community health services.

Professional Standards Review

The advent of professional standards review poses still another opportunity for the planner. Sooner or later, care delivered in emergency departments will be subjected to such review. While standards may be developed by specialists in national programs, their application to quality assessment in local areas requires adaptive mechanisms that can be developed by health planners in cooperation with medical personnel. In addition to monitoring and assessing the quality of the process of emergency care, there is an opportunity to develop methods for following patients to determine the outcomes of this care. This determination is crucial to assessment of the overall impact of investments made in the emergency system. This little explored area offers unusual opportunities for development.

THE EMERGENCY SYSTEM OUTSIDE THE HOSPITAL

Outside the hospital, attention must be given to the components of the emergency system that bring the patient to the emergency department. A health emergency occurs when someone perceives a condition that requires urgent medical care. It is this perception that initiates the chain of events. If the perceptions of the man in the street are not adequate or if he lacks the knowledge to activate the system effectively, the results are bound to be less than desirable, no matter how sophisticated the system may be. Once an urgent situation is perceived, communication linkages must be available and a response system must be ready and capable of rapid arrival and appropriate action at the site of the event.

From the point of view of the planner, this involves consideration of many factors: the communication linkages; the training and knowledge of the dispatchers; the location, personnel, and equipment of the emergency response units; and the methods by which the decisions are made regarding onsite action and transport. Finally, the direction of the patient to an appropriate facility requires a plan for categorization of hospitals, and the authority to make such decisions. There may be a necessity for two-way radio communication and consultation among the dispatching center, the hospital, and the squads in the field. The planner may have to serve as an evaluator and even as a pro-tem system manager. It is very difficult for planning agencies to divorce themselves completely from the implementation phase of such critical services.

EMTs

In general, there is a low level of competition in most aspects of emergency services. Physicians do not leave their offices to seek emergencies, and hospital personnel rarely leave their facilities. If they would, it would indeed be an inefficient use of such personnel. Consequently, this area has become open for the innovative use of new types of health personnel.

The development of the EMT is a prime example of the innovation. There is no other aspect of the health-care system in which nonphysicians have been given so much responsibility away from the immediate supervision of physicians. Well-trained EMTs have proved their capabilities in administering vital and critical care to patients with serious illness and injury away from the hospital and beyond the reach of medical supervision. Their success opens the door to consideration of specific task-oriented assignments for other paramedical personnel that may extend a variety of health-care services to the overall population and maximize the service capacity of the physician. The physician then has the unusual opportunity to concentrate on the more complex aspects of health care, synthesizing clinical information and developing new approaches to the prevention of disease, the maintenance of health, and treatment of illness at a higher level of scientific application.

Employee First-Aid Training

The Occupational Safety and Health Act poses still another possibility for the planner. One of the standards of this act involves availability of first-aid to all employees in their places of work. There is need for initiative in providing appropriate educational programs to the workers. Each employer can arrange for an appropriate number of employees to receive such education. Once trained they can be deployed throughout the place of work, so that at least one is available to take critical action at each site on each shift. The trained workers would be responsible for communication with the local emergency squads and the initiation of appropriate actions at the site prior to their arrival. This process will augment the number of individuals in the community educated in emergency matters and may thus enhance emergency services in sparsely served areas. By arrangements with local volunteer groups or public ambulance services, workers who are specially trained in first-aid can work with the emergency squads at arranged times to augment the services and to keep their own skills fresh. The health planner and his agency thus have an opportunity to interact with local commercial and industrial organizations and to inform them of the overall health status and health needs of the community. These organizations are a powerful constituency in health planning.

Emergency Response System

The prehospital emergency response system is usually made up of a loose agglomeration of personnel, vehicles, and equipment, with varying degrees of capability. In many areas, the emergency response system is still the province of the funeral director or of a rudimentary volunteer service. Such organizations deliver vital services in areas where no other emergency service exists. It would be unwise to force the elimination of such services without first providing an alternative. However, it is dangerous to have a system with services of various levels of capability. It is likely that the more rudimentary services will force the more sophisticated and more expensive services out of the market. This situation can be remedied by setting uniform standards, such as those developed by the U.S. Department of Transportation, and working out a plan for the implementation of service to meet these standards in a given region. This process may take time and public and private investments. The vast majority of emergency services are devoted to delivery of adequate service, however, and with the appropriate encouragement and assistance, even the most remote areas can attain services of minimum essential quality.

THE PLANNING PROCESS

In general, the planning of emergency medical services is not unlike the planning of other medical services, but the factor of presumed urgency offers special advantages. It is possible to play the "pin-in-the-map" game as a start of planning. By pinpointing any spot in the region for which the planning is being done, the planner may collect data to determine the incidence of specific emergency events in that area. The determination would, of course, be conditioned by demographic variables and the presence of agents or opportunities for the occurrence of emergencies. On the basis of such determinations, the planner may ask what would happen to an individual with a particular problem at that spot? What is the likelihood that need for emergency care would be recognized? How would communication be made with the emergency system? Who would respond? What would be the capabilities of the response? How long would it take? What could be done at the site of the event? Where would the patient be transported? What would be the capabilities in the receiving emergency department? What provisions would there be for transfer to centers with specialized capabilities?

This "game" can highlight the status of the area, its needs, and the gaps that exist in the current system. On this basis, objectives can be set, and the series of alternative approaches to these objectives can be developed. These objectives can be stated in terms of time, necessary resources, and likelihood of accomplishment.

The opportunities for the health planner in emergency health care are clearly present and somewhat unique. They combine the possibility of an early demonstration of results, a high likelihood of success, and a wide area of impact on vital community needs. This opportunity is a combination difficult to beat and a challenge difficult to resist.

Appendixes

Appendix A

A Check List for Airport Disaster Planning: The Medical Annex

		Yes	No

I. Purpose: Does the plan indicate the purpose of providing emergency services? ___ ___
—care for the emergency needs of air travelers and airport employees? ___ ___
—disaster medical care? ___ ___
—aid and assistance to uninjured survivors? ___ ___
—cooperation with disaster agencies of local communities? ___ ___

II. Authorities: Does the plan cite the appropriate laws and regulations requiring emergency preparedness? ___ ___
—federal, state, and local laws governing responsibilities? ___ ___
—regulations for certification and operation of land airports serving CAB-certified air carriers and Part 139.55 of Federal Aviation Regulations (FAA)? ___ ___
—incorporation within airport operator's emergency plan? ___ ___
—incorporation with the community disaster plan? ___ ___

III. Policies: Does the plan describe basic humanitarian responsibilities as approved by the airport operator? ___ ___
—extent and limitation of disaster medical services rendered? ___ ___
—welfare services for uninjured survivors? ___ ___

—transfer and transportation responsibilities for
survivors? ⎯ ⎯
—airline and other tenant responsibilities? ⎯ ⎯
IV. Scope: Does the plan describe the extent and
limitations of emergency and disaster services? ⎯ ⎯
—extent of authority to provide services at or near
airport? ⎯ ⎯
—cooperation and coordination with airport and
community agencies? ⎯ ⎯
—training and continuing education of health
personnel? ⎯ ⎯
V. Definitions: Does the plan clearly define the
elements that relate to medical emergencies? ⎯ ⎯
—emergency medical services? ⎯ ⎯
—aircraft accident or incident? ⎯ ⎯
—aircraft disaster? ⎯ ⎯
—triage and casualty sorting procedures? ⎯ ⎯
—disaster medical services? ⎯ ⎯
—medical authority and command? ⎯ ⎯
VI. Notification and alerting procedures: Does the
plan clearly indicate a cascade system and
alternatives for notification with certain types of
disasters or emergencies? ⎯ ⎯
—aircraft incidents and accidents? ⎯ ⎯
—aircraft disasters? ⎯ ⎯
—bomb, sabotage, and highjacking incidents? ⎯ ⎯
—airport fires and explosions? ⎯ ⎯
—natural disasters? ⎯ ⎯
—radiological or nuclear incidents? ⎯ ⎯
VII. Primary and secondary agency alerts: Does the
plan clearly identify the alerting of the following? ⎯ ⎯
—disaster medical director? ⎯ ⎯
—airport medical facility staff (roster)? ⎯ ⎯
—disaster medical team(s)? ⎯ ⎯
—community, military, Veterans Administration,
and other hospitals? ⎯ ⎯
—ambulance services (air, ground, water)? ⎯ ⎯
—medical examiner or coroner's office? ⎯ ⎯
—disaster medical service elements of
airline medical office? ⎯ ⎯
civil defense? ⎯ ⎯
Red Cross? ⎯ ⎯

health department?   —— ——

hospital council?   —— ——

county medical society?   —— ——

—Search and Rescue Division, U.S. Coast Guard
Operations Office?   —— ——

—Funeral Director's Association?   —— ——

VIII. Roles and responsibilities: Does the plan clearly
define the responsibilities of key personnel?   —— ——

—emergency medical teams?   —— ——

—ambulance services?   —— ——

—fire and rescue services (first responders)?   —— ——

IX. Disaster communications and operations centers
for medical operations: Does the plan indicate the
radio and other communication systems available
to the disaster medical director, ambulances, and
hospitals?   —— ——

—airport disaster headquarters?   —— ——

—disaster site command post?   —— ——

X. Disaster site emergency care: Does the plan
indicate or describe the following:

—casualty collecting point?   —— ——

—sorting principles?   —— ——

—triage coding system?   —— ——

—extent and limitations of emergency care?   —— ——

—management of the dead?   —— ——

—a grid map of the airport with best locations for
establishing emergency medical operations?   —— ——

—records and tagging procedures?   —— ——

—weather protection?   —— ——

—lighting and night operation?   —— ——

—special equipment and supplies?   —— ——

XI. Mobile or stationary casualty support facility: Do
the needs of disaster services require a holding
ward or medical facility at the airport?   —— ——

—conditions of activation?   —— ——

—location and staffing?   —— ——

—storage of equipment and supplies (refurbishing
and upkeep)?   —— ——

XII. Off-airport disasters: Does the plan include or
explain roles of airport emergency operations and
staff when accidents occur in the local community?   —— ——

—agreements with local governmental and medical
disaster authorities?   —— ——

—definition of responsible disaster medical
director? ___ ___
—description of procedures and operations? ___ ___

XIII. Records and information services: Does the plan
provide for records on all casualties and
noncasualty survivors at the disaster site? ___ ___
—name or other identification? ___ ___
—condition on rescue? ___ ___
—treatment and disposition? ___ ___
—directions on release of information by medical
personnel to the authorities and news media? ___ ___

XIV. Training programs, drills, and rehearsals: Does a
regular program exist for
—training and education of
physicians? ___ ___
nurses? ___ ___
EMTs? ___ ___
fire fighters? ___ ___
other airport personnel? ___ ___
—policies on maintenance of disaster skills? ___ ___
—disaster rehearsal
frequency? ___ ___
critiques (preparation and distribution)? ___ ___
rewriting plans? ___ ___
annual report to all concerned on readiness status? ___ ___

Appendix B

State of Michigan
Senate Bill No. 987

June 18, 1975. Introduced by Senators Otterbacher, Faxon, Cartwright, Bursley, De Grow, and Holmes and referred to the Committee on Health, Social Services, and Retirement.

A bill to provide for the development of an emergency medical services system; to impose certain duties upon the department of public health and other state agencies; to provide for the creation of a state-wide emergency medical services advisory committee; and to provide for the creation of regional emergency medical services advisory committees.

THE PEOPLE OF THE STATE OF MICHIGAN ENACT

Sec. 1. This act shall be known and may be cited as the "emergency medical service system act of 1975."

Sec. 2. As used in this act

(a) *Ambulance* means a vehicle that is used or designated as routinely available to provide transportation or transportation and treatment for patients and is authorized as part of a licensed ambulance operation by the department pursuant to Act No. 258 of the Public Acts of 1968, as amended, being sections 257.1201 to 257.1217 of Michigan Compiled Laws.

(b) *Ambulance operation* means a person, firm, partnership, association, corporation, company, group of individuals, or a government agency licensed by the department to provide, whether for profit or otherwise, the licensed personnel, ambulances, and other equipment required to transport and render emergency medical services to patients.

(c) *Consumer* means a resident of the state who is a recipient or potential recipient of the services provided by an emergency medical services system, who receives no direct or indirect personal, financial,

337

or professional benefit as a result of an association with health care or emergency services other than that generally shared by the public at large, and who is not otherwise considered a provider under the terms and conditions of this act.

(d) *Department* means the Michigan department of public health.

(e) *Designated regional health planning agency* means a health systems agency created pursuant to Public Law 93–641 known as the national health planning and resource development act of 1974, or a regional comprehensive health planning agency created pursuant to 42 U.S.C. section 246(b), as amended.

(f) *Director* means the director of the Michigan department of public health.

(g) *Emergency medical services system* means a comprehensive and integrated arrangement of all personnel, facilities, equipment, services, and organizations necessary to provide emergency medical treatment to patients.

(h) *Emergency medical technician* means an individual who has completed a department approved emergency medical technician ambulance course prescribed by the United States department of transportation or an equivalent course approved by the department, and who is licensed by the department pursuant to Act No. 275 of the Public Acts of 1974, as amended.

(i) *Patient* means an individual who as a result of illness or injury needs immediate medical attention, whose physical or mental condition is such that he is in imminent danger of loss of life or significant health impairment, or who may be otherwise incapacitated or helpless as a result of a physical or mental condition.

(j) *Provider* means a person or the spouse of a person who, as an individual or member of a corporation or organization, whether profit or nonprofit, on a regular basis gives or offers for sale any supplies, equipment, professional or nonprofessional service, or is capable of giving or offering for sale supplies, equipment, or professional services vital for the provision of an organized emergency medical service system.

Sec. 3. The department shall

(a) Be responsible for the planning, coordination, and administration of a state-wide emergency medical services system.

(b) Annually inventory or cause to be inventoried emergency medical services resources within the state for the purposes of determining the need for additional services and the effectiveness of existing services.

(c) Develop a standardized planning format for regional planning activities.

(d) Review, evaluate, and integrate all regional emergency medical services plans developed by the designated regional health planning agencies pursuant to section 6 of this act in order to prepare a state-wide emergency medical services plan. The state-wide plan shall contain (i) a statement of specific measurable objectives for the delivery of emergency medical services; (ii) the methods used to achieve the objectives; (iii) a schedule for achievement of the objectives; and (iv) a method for evaluating the objectives.

(e) Update the state-wide plan for the coordinated delivery of emergency medical services at least every 3 years.

(f) Develop and administer a state-wide data collection system based on standardized forms and procedures. The state-wide data collection system shall include uniform patient records which will follow a patient from initial entry into the emergency medical service system through discharge from treatment programs, and shall provide for the development of other data necessary for evaluation.

(g) Evaluate the availability and quality of emergency medical care to assure a reasonable standard of performance by individuals and organizations providing such services.

(h) Develop and conduct a program of public information and education relating to emergency medical services.

(i) Develop an emergency medical services plan for a region in the event that no plan is submitted by a designated regional health planning agency pursuant to section 6 of this act. The plan shall conform to the requirements of section 6.

(j) Within 45 days of their receipt, review and comment on all grant and contract applications for federal, state, or private funds concerning emergency medical services or related activities, and forward those applications to the appropriate agency. An application not acted on by the department within 45 days shall be considered reviewed and favorably commented on.

(k) In the event of disaster, assume command and control of emergency medical services and related transportation and communications operations consistent with the Michigan emergency preparedness plan.

(l) Consistent with the rules of the federal communications commission, coordinate the development and assure the integration of the state-wide radio communications facilities network for emergency medical services.

(m) Promulgate rules in accordance with the intent of this act pursuant to Act No. 306 of the Public Acts of 1969, as amended, being sections 24.201 to 24.315 of the Michigan Compiled Laws.

Sec. 4. (1) There shall be established within the department a state-wide emergency medical service advisory committee which shall be composed of 19 members. The committee shall include three emergency physicians, one of whom shall be a doctor of osteopathy. There shall be one representative of each of the following groups: (a) fire officials; (b) law enforcement officials; (c) hospitals; (d) ambulance associations; (e) emergency nurses; and (f) emergency medical technicians. Ten members shall be consumers. At least one consumer shall be appointed from each regional emergency medical service advisory committee established in section 7 of this act.

(2) State agencies and private, nonprofit service agencies may participate as *ex officio* members of the committee.

(3) At least one provider member shall be appointed from each regional emergency medical service advisory committee. All provider members will be recommended to the governor by the Michigan emergency services health council.

(4) All members of the committee shall be appointed by the governor with the advice and consent of the senate. Of the members first appointed, ten members shall be appointed for a term of 2 years, and nine for 3 years. Thereafter, members shall be appointed for a term of 3 years.

(5) The *per diem* for the state-wide emergency medical services advisory committee members and a schedule for reimbursement of expenses shall be established annually by the legislature.

(6) Eleven members shall constitute a quorum for the transaction of business, six of whom shall be consumers. The chairperson shall be a consumer elected annually from the committee. The committee shall meet at least four times annually at the call of the chairperson or the director. All meetings of the committee shall be open to the public.

Sec. 5. The state-wide emergency medical service advisory committee shall

(a) Approve or disapprove the proposed state plan created pursuant to section 3 (d).

(b) Advise the department on a standardized planning format pursuant to section 3 (c).

(c) Advise the department on the development of a state-wide data collection system pursuant to section 3 (f).

(d) Advise the department on the development of a program of public information and education pursuant to section 3 (h).

(e) Advise the director concerning the categorization of emergency facilities and services pursuant to section 5 of Act No. 17 of the Public Acts of 1968, being section 331.415 of the Michigan Compiled Laws.

Sec. 6. (1) The designated regional health-planning agencies shall be the regional planning and coordinating agencies for emergency medical services and shall provide continuous evaluation of emergency medical services for their respective geographic areas and shall report their evaluations to the department. The agencies shall annually develop and submit to the department a plan for the delivery of emergency medical services. The plan shall be consistent with the policies established for the state-wide emergency medical service system and shall include

(a) A statement of specific measurable objectives for the delivery of emergency medical services.

(b) Methods used to achieve the objectives.

(c) A schedule for methods used to achieve the objectives.

(d) Estimated cost for attaining the methods used to achieve the objectives.

(e) Performance standards for evaluation of the objectives.

(f) Provisions for but not be limited to (i) clearly defined geographical regions to be served by each ambulance operation including cooperative arrangements with other providers and backup services; (ii) an adequate number of trained personnel for staffing of ambulances, communication facilities, hospital emergency rooms, and other emergency related services; (iii) acquisition of necessary emergency equipment; (iv) a communications system that includes a central dispatch center, a central emergency resource coordination facility, links to the state-wide emergency medical radio network, 2-way radio communication between the ambulance and the receiving hospital, and a universal emergency telephone number, when such a number is appropriate; (v) a public education program that stresses appropriate utilization of the emergency medical services system for that region, basic lifesaving techniques, and other necessary information.

(2) The agency shall perform its functions in cooperation with each appropriate regional emergency medical services advisory committee as established by section 7 and shall provide necessary staff assistance to the regional emergency medical services advisory committee.

(3) The agency shall delegate to such local organizations as are willing to accept the responsibility, the responsibility for local emergency medical services planning and shall assist local organizations to develop a plan that will include the components enumerated in Public Law 93-154, being 42 U.S.C. sections 300d, *et seq.* The plan shall deal with the subjects of: (i) manpower; (ii) training; (iii) communications; (iv) transportation; (v) facilities; (vi) critical care units; (vii) public safety agencies; (viii) consumer participation; (ix) accessibility to care; (x) transfer of patients; (xi) standard medical record-keeping; (xii) evaluation; (xiii) disaster linkage; (xiv) mutual aid agreements; and (xv) consumer information and education.

(4) The agency shall forward all grant and contract applications to the department at least 45 days prior to the initiation of the funding agency's review process.

Sec. 7. In each designated health-planning region, there shall be established a regional emergency medical service advisory committee. Opportunity for membership shall be available to all appropriate representatives from, but not limited to, each of the following: (a) local governments; (b) fire officials; (c) law enforcement officials; (d) emergency physicians; (e) emergency care nurses; (f) mental health professionals; (g) emergency medical technicians; (h) allied health professionals; (i) providers of ambulance services, including both paid and volunteer services; (j) hospitals. Consumers shall comprise at least 51% of the total number of committee members. All emergency medical service advisory committees shall submit to the department information concerning the organizational structure and committee bylaws. All committee meetings shall be open to the public. The regional emergency medical services committee members shall be appointed by the designated regional health planning agency.

Sec. 8. Each regional emergency medical service advisory committee shall

(a) Approve or disapprove within 45 days the regional health-planning agency's plan.

(b) Approve or disapprove the designated regional health planning agency's policies and priorities regarding emergency medical services.

(c) Approve or disapprove within 45 days the designated regional health-planning agency's recommendations regarding all grant and contract applications for federal and state funds pertaining to emergency medical services.

Sec. 9. Each designated regional health-planning agency shall have a regional emergency medical services coordinator who shall be appointed by the designated regional health-planning agency.

Sec. 10. The regional emergency medical services coordinator shall be responsible to the designated regional health-planning agency for (a) facilitating the work of the designated regional health-planning agency and the department in developing the plan for the coordination of emergency medical services within the region; (b) assisting in implementation of the regional plan formulated by the designated regional health planning agency pursuant to section 6; (c) continuous monitoring and evaluation of all emergency medical services in that region; and (d) making a complete inventory of all personnel, facilities, and equipment within the region related to the delivery of emergency medical services.

Sec. 11. (1) All state agencies shall to the fullest extent of their authority under state law administer programs under their control in such a manner as to further the establishment of coordinated, state-wide emergency medical services system.

(2) All state agencies shall cooperate with the department, the state-wide emergency medical services advisory committee, the designated regional health planning agencies, regional emergency medical service coordinators, and regional emergency medical services advisory committees in developing the state emergency medical services program under this act.

(3) All state agencies concerned with the state-wide emergency medical services system shall cooperate with the appropriate agencies of the United States, or of other states, or interstate and Canadian agencies with respect to the planning, coordination, and implementation of emergency medical services.

Sec. 12. Nothing in this act shall be construed to deny emergency medical services to persons outside the boundaries of the state of Michigan nor shall this act be construed so as to limit, restrict, or prevent any cooperative agreement for the provision of emergency medical services between the state of Michigan, or any of its political subunits, and any of the other United States or federal agencies, or their political subunits, or the Dominion of Canada or its political subunits.

Sec. 13. The attorney general, a political subdivision of the state, an instrumentality or agency of the state or of a political subdivision thereof, a person, partnership, corporation, association, organization, or other legal entity may maintain an action in the circuit court for declaratory and equitable relief against the department or designated regional health-planning agency to enforce this act or the rules promulgated pursuant to this act. Costs may be apportioned to the parties as the interests of justice require. Nothing in this act shall apply to any service, facility, or equipment owned and operated by an agency or department of the United States government unless that service, facility, or equipment is integrated into the state-wide emergency medical services system. A private person, but not a governmental agency, who brings and prevails in a suit under this section may recover reasonable attorney's fees.

Sec. 14. This act shall take effect July 1, 1976.